Compassionate Communities

Compassionate communities are communities that provide assistance for those in need of end-of-life care, separate from any official heath service provision that may already be available within the community. This idea was developed in 2005 in Allan Kellehear's seminal volume *Compassionate Cities: Public health and end-of-life care*. In the ensuing ten years the theoretical aspects of the idea have been continually explored, primarily rehearsing academic concerns rather than practical ones.

Compassionate Communities: Case studies from Britain and Europe provides the first major volume describing and examining compassionate community experiments in end-of-life care from a highly practical perspective. Focusing on community development initiatives and practice challenges, the book offers practitioners and policy makers from the health and social care sectors practical discussions on the strengths and limitations of such initiatives. Furthermore, not limited to providing practice choices the book also offers an important and timely impetus for other practitioners and policy makers to begin thinking about developing their own possible compassionate communities.

An essential read for academic, practitioner, and policy audiences in the fields of public health, community development, health social sciences, aged care, bereavement care, and hospice and palliative care, *Compassionate Communities* is one of only a handful of available books on end-of-life care that takes a strong health promotion and community development approach.

Klaus Wegleitner is Assistant Professor, Institute of Palliative Care and Organisational Ethics, Faculty of Interdisciplinary Studies (IFF Vienna), Alpen-Adria University Klagenfurt, Vienna, Austria.

Katharina Heimerl is Associate Professor and Head, Institute of Palliative Care and Organisational Ethics, Faculty of Interdisciplinary Studies (IFF Vienna), Alpen-Adria University Klagenfurt, Vienna, Austria.

Allan Kellehear is 50th Anniversary Chair – Professor of End-of-Life Care, University of Bradford, UK.

Routledge Key Themes in Health and Society

Available titles include:

Turning Troubles into Problems
Clientization in Human Services
Edited by Jaber F. Gubrium and Margaretha Järvinen

Compassionate Communities
Case Studies from Britain and Europe
Edited by Klaus Wegleitner, Katharina Heimerl and Allan Kellehear

Forthcoming titles include:

Empowerment: A Critique
Written by Kenneth McLaughlin

Exploring Evidence-based Practice
Edited by Martin Lipscomb

Living with Mental Disorder
Insights from Qualitative Research
Written by Jacqueline Corcoran

The Politics of Ignorance in Nursing and Healthcare
Written by Amélie Perron and Trudy Rudge

Compassionate Communities
Case studies from Britain and Europe

Edited by Klaus Wegleitner,
Katharina Heimerl and Allan Kellehear

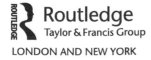

Routledge
Taylor & Francis Group

LONDON AND NEW YORK

First published 2016
by Routledge
2 Park Square, Milton Park, Abingdon, Oxon OX14 4RN

and by Routledge
711 Third Avenue, New York, NY 10017

First issued in paperback 2017

Routledge is an imprint of the Taylor & Francis Group, an informa business

British Library Cataloguing-in-Publication Data
A catalogue record for this book is available from the British Library

Library of Congress Cataloging in Publication Data
Compassionate communities : case studies from Britain and Europe / edited by Klaus Wegleitner, Katharina Heimerl, and Allan Kellehear.
p. ; cm. -- (Routledge key themes in health and society)
Includes bibliographical references.
I. Wegleitner, Klaus, editor. II. Heimerl, Katharina, editor. III. Kellehear, Allan, 1955- , editor. IV. Series: Routledge key themes in health and society.
[DNLM: 1. Community Health Services--organization & administration. 2. Terminal Care--organization & administration. 3. Community Health Planning--organization & administration. 4. Empathy. 5. Palliative Care--organization & administration. 6. Public Policy. WB 310]
R726.8
362.17'56--dc23
2014048611

ISBN 13: 978-1-138-55203-6 (pbk)
ISBN 13: 978-1-138-83279-4 (hbk)

Typeset in Sabon
by Saxon Graphics Ltd, Derby

Contents

Figures

Figures

Contributors

Julian Abel is Medical Consultant in Palliative Care, Weston Hospicecare and Weston Area Health Trust, UK.

Antonia Bunnin is Director of Hospice Support and Development, Hospice UK, London, UK.

Paul Cronin is Chief Executive, Severn Hospice, Shrewsbury, Shropshire, UK.

Reimer Gronemeyer is Professor of Sociology, Justus-Liebig University, Gießen, Germany.

Katharina Heimerl is Associate Professor and Head, Institute of Palliative Care and Organizational Ethics, Faculty of Interdisciplinary Studies (IFF Vienna), Alpen-Adria University Klagenfurt, Vienna, Austria.

Andreas Heller is Professor of Palliative Care and Organizational Ethics, IFF Vienna, Alpen-Adria University Klagenfurt, Vienna, Austria.

Siobhan Horton is Director of Clinical Services, St Luke's Cheshire Hospice, Winsford, Cheshire, UK.

Karin Kaspers-Elekes is Commissioner for Palliative Care, Evangelical Church of Thurgau, Chair Palliative Care Network Eastern Switzerland 'palliative ostschweiz', St. Gallen, Switzerland.

Allan Kellehear is 50th Anniversary Chair – Professor of End-of-Life Care, University of Bradford, UK.

Thomas Klie is Professor of Public Law and Administrative Sciences, Protestant University of Applied Sciences, Head of Center for Developments in Civil Society, Freiburg, Germany.

Katharina Linsi is Lecturer at the Educational Center for Health and Social Affairs, Head of Palliative Care, Weidenfeld, Member Executive Board at palliative ostschweiz, Rheineck, Switzerland.

Kathleen McLoughlin is All Ireland Institute of Hospice and Palliative Care and Irish Cancer Society Research Fellow, Department of Psychology, Maynooth University and Compassionate Communities Project Co-ordinator, Milford Care Centre, Limerick, Ireland.

Bie Nio Ong is Professor of Health Services Research, Keele University, UK.

Manjula Patel is Health Services Manager, Bridges Support Service, Murray Hall Community Trust, Oldbury, West Midlands, UK.

Petra Plunger is Community Pharmacist and Researcher, Institute of Palliative Care and Organizational Ethics, IFF Vienna, Alpen-Adria University Klagenfurt, Vienna, Austria.

Sonja Prieth is Researcher at the IFF Vienna, Alpen-Adria University Klagenfurt, Vienna, Austria, and Head of Education, Tyrolean Hospice Association, Innsbruck, Austria.

Elisabeth Reitinger is Associate Professor, Institute of Palliative Care and Organizational Ethics, IFF Vienna, Alpen-Adria University Klagenfurt, Vienna, Austria.

Jim Rhatigan is Head of Therapies and Social Care, Milford Care Centre, Limerick, Ireland.

Heather Richardson is Joint Chief Executive, St Christopher's Hospice, London, and Compassionate Communities Adviser, St Joseph's Hospice, London, UK.

Verena Rothe is Executive Director, Aktion Demenz, Gießen, Germany.

Libby Sallnow is a palliative medicine registrar and research fellow at St Joseph's Hospice, London, and a doctoral student at the University of Edinburgh, UK.

Patrick Schuchter is Researcher and Lecturer, Institute of Palliative Care and Organizational Ethics, IFF Vienna, Alpen-Adria University Klagenfurt, Vienna, Austria.

Verena Tatzer is Researcher and Lecturer, IFF Vienna, Alpen-Adria University Klagenfurt, Vienna, Austria, and at the University of Applied Sciences Wiener Neustadt, Austria.

Ditch Townsend is Compassionate Communities Network Co-ordinator, Weston Hospicecare, UK.

Elisabeth Wappelshammer is Researcher and Lecturer, Institute of Palliative Care and Organizational Ethics, IFF Vienna, Alpen-Adria University Klagenfurt, Vienna, Austria.

Klaus Wegleitner is Assistant Professor, Institute of Palliative Care and Organizational Ethics, IFF Vienna, Alpen-Adria University Klagenfurt, Vienna, Austria.

Christine Weissenberg is Psychiatrist and Psychotherapist, Bern, Switzerland.

Rachel Zammit is Head of Public Health and Wellbeing, End of Life Partnership, Cheshire, UK.

Preface

Although the idea that whole cities, towns and villages should be subject to public health policies and practices has been embraced for centuries, with the latest developments embodied in the World Health Organization's (WHO) 'healthy cities' movement, the application of these kinds of ideas into community experiences of dying, death, loss and end of life care is only recent. It is also true that most traditional communities have long had policies on the disposal of the dead and community support of the dying, bereaved and their caregivers. However, most modern communities have had the last of these cultural norms of support gradually eroded through their historical re-(dis-)placement by professional and government services. Indeed, the massive development of a health and social services infrastructure in the twentieth century has led to a widespread deskilling of communities in relation to dying, bereavement and caregiving in particular.

To counter, repair and reconstruct some of these lost skills in community health maintenance and care the health promotion and community development movement – within public health, social work, pastoral care and international development – has aspired to combine modern health knowledge and services with local community knowledge and social action. To meet the ideals of prevention, harm reduction and early intervention in modern public health it was widely recognized by most modern governments that these can only be attained in partnership with the local citizenry. People need to learn or relearn how to help themselves. The reason for this principle of self-help is not related to the recent health policy cynicism of 'cost-savings' and 'cost-rationalizations' that might assist with diminishing or poor healthcare budgets but rather and most importantly because even the best health care cannot be everywhere at all times. Continuity and optimal quality of care is only possible by way of a partnership between formal services and the communities that surround and support individuals and families. Even the most responsive health and social care service will be episodic – it cannot be a constant and close-by presence, a constant and close-by helping hand, a constant and close-by companion. Moreover, some problems – such as loneliness, stigma, social rejection or caregiver fatigue – are not most effectively addressed by professionals or services.

Compassionate communities are communities that develop social networks, social spaces, social policies and social conduct that support people through the many hours, days, weeks, months and sometimes years of living with a life-threatening or life-limiting illness, ageing, grief and bereavement, and long-term caregiving. They do this through organization and deployment of volunteers, or through the creation of policies (public expectations) in workplaces or schools to shape supportive responses. They may also adopt public charters for social action, or they may create or modify professional services so that these services facilitate, foster and build community engagement that may eventually lead to culture change – from individualist cultures of isolated families with their own networks, to communalist cultures that foster outreach between neighbours, parishioners or business colleagues and school friends. Compassionate communities are an expression of shared values and fundamental ethical attitudes, such as empathy, mindfulness, attentiveness, respect and solidarity in human coexistence. They are seeking for ways for how caring responsibilities in societies might be distributed and assigned democratically (consistent with the values of social justice, equity and freedom) and also to ensure the greatest possible participation of citizens in this assignment of responsibilities. They are modern health communities that believe that not only is health everyone's business but also the journey at the end of life itself. Care at the end of life is not simply a professional or services matter, nor is it a matter of good fortune or serendipity but rather a conscious, planned and deliberate political and social set of actions taken by the key players in any community to enhance the support and wellbeing of everyone affected by ageing, dying, death, loss and caregiving.

This book is a collection of case studies to show how different communities in Europe have attempted to create the first compassionate communities. They have drawn broadly for their inspiration, sometimes from general community development theory (Minkler and Wallerstein, 2008), sometimes specifically from Suresh Kumar's (2007) Neighbourhood Network ideas or Allan Kellehear's (2005) Compassionate Cities ideas, sometimes from the model of social action embraced by the 'dementia-friendly communities' social movement, or the concept of a caring culture in the third social space (Dörner, 2007).

Whatever the source of their inspiration, all of the models showcased in this book are attempting to move their professional and service practices from community-based services (working on directing, influencing and servicing people in their community setting) to community engagement (working with and alongside communities in *joint* actions and decisions) and toward community development (communities taking major responsibility in determining their own end of life care needs and developing means for addressing them). Care is a right we expect not only from the State and its representatives *but also from each other*.

We hope that this volume will be read and used not only by students but also by practitioners, policy makers and academics in public health, social and spiritual care, international development, local government, and end of life care. And by 'end of life care' we mean the broadest array of those normally engaged in this field: from palliative care, pastoral care, care of older people, dementia care and bereavement care – to others working in disaster management, intensive care, accident and emergency care, veterinarian science, and funeral care. Our aim is to show real-time experiments shaped by the exigencies of local culture, pressures and limitations. We want to show that compassionate communities are achievable social practices – not simply 'idealistic', romantic or sentimental constructions. Although compassionate communities are characterized by a diverse set of approaches and methods they are all underpinned by a core set of social and public health values despite this diversity: strengthening social cohesion and self-help resources, enhancement of wellbeing at the end of life, addressing the social epidemiology of ageing, dying, death, loss and caregiving – together as a community, and working to address the gaps in quality and continuity of care at the end of life.

Chapter 1 takes a broad overview of the compassionate communities movement in the United Kingdom (UK) tracing its roots to volunteering and community development sources. This chapter also examines the challenges facing hospices and palliative care services in particular that desire to embrace community development. Chapter 2 describes a specific compassionate community project in Weston-super-Mare in England tracing its roots to inspiration from different sources of academic and practice work from Australia. Chapter 3 similarly describes a compassionate community project in Shropshire in England – also based from a hospice – and presents some of the first solid and impressive evaluation evidence for its effectiveness. Chapter 4 describes the establishment of a compassionate community project from community organization whose main brief is social rather than clinical care. This chapter showcases an important practice example from an organization that has no major connection with the UK hospice movement. Chapter 5 looks specifically at how one hospice creates a partnership-based approach towards working with communities to share responsibility for end of life care. This chapter describes its blended approach toward education, advocacy, community engagement and service provision. Chapter 6 describes a community charter used to invite the social and cultural sectors of community to participate in end of life care. The charter identifies sectors and actions that key community players can take to enhance end of life care in their community. Chapter 7 describes the first compassionate community experiments from the Republic of Ireland. This chapter also showcases its particular blend of education, advocacy, community engagement and service provision but also illustrates its use of social media in communicating this new message of community participation. Chapter 8 describes a 'caring community' experiment in Austria illustrating the blend of action research and policy and practice implementation in partnership with local community sectors of government, informal and professional caregivers, self-help groups, schools, engaged citizens and other key players within that community. The contribution of building compassionate communities to the complementary idea of 'caring society' is also discussed. Chapter 9 showcases a specific approach to compassionate communities whose emphasis is specifically on the development of empathy between community members through shared narratives of care and concern. It is argued that only through the development of genuine empathy can genuine care be offered. The chapter outlines a paradigmatic shift from clinical ethics to 'communal' ethics. Chapter 10 examines the role of the community pharmacy in providing and enhancing community support for people living with dementia. Methods used to provide informal support for people living with dementia and their caregivers are outlined. Measures that contribute to decrease stigmatization are performed by the pharmacies. Chapter 11 describes a study of end of life care in a Swiss convent. This chapter examines the minute interpersonal behaviours and experiences of care between the resident nuns and between the nuns and the wider community in caring for their frail elderly in particular. Conclusions are drawn with respect to 'caring democracy' (Tronto, 2013) and the potentials of translating pre-professional forms of supportive cultures into the practice of contemporary end of life care in the community. Chapter 12 describes the setting up of local palliative care forums as part of a community network in end of life care in Eastern Switzerland based on the earlier work in Kerala, India. The emphasis here is on the specific role of forums in strengthening very local care arrangements and enabling negotiations over basic ethical and cultural principles in the community. Chapter 13 introduces the dementia-friendly community movement in Germany. This chapter shows how well community development models can work for specific groups such as the elderly with dementia. Experiences from the nationwide funding programme 'People in the Community Living with Dementia' are critically analysed. Finally, Chapter 14 looks broadly at the problem and meaning of the two key terms of 'caring' and 'community' in the context of German society. How these terms are interpreted, what controversies they trigger and how the concepts are made real in Germany is the focus of this discussion.

All these chapters describe the practical detail of their different efforts but all do so with a close eye on the challenges and difficulties they faced as well as reflections on the future of their attempts. The chapters are written collegially, that is, with the intention of sharing practical experience and reflection with colleagues among our readership who wish to take the same direction but lack colleagues to talk with about their aspirations and plans. By reading the following chapters newcomers can benefit from the practice-wisdom inherent in the trail-blazing experiments within these pages whilst others already involved with these kinds of approaches may gain further support and additional insight in continuing their important work. For without our own 'community' to share and develop with and alongside we cannot hope to ask the same of others. We must model the meaning of participation and cooperation in community and it is within that spirit that this book is written and offered.

KW, KH and AK
Jointly in Vienna, Austria, and Bradford, England
2014

References

Dörner, K. (2007) *Leben und sterben, wo ich hingehöre. Dritter Sozialraum und neues Hilfesystem* (To live and to die, where I belong. Third Social Space and new Help System). Neumünster: Paranus-Verlag.

Kellehear, A. (2005) *Compassionate Cites: Public Health and End-of-Life Care.* London: Routledge.

Kumer, S. (2007) Kerala, India: a regional community-based palliative care model. *Journal of Pain and Symptom Management* 33(5): 623–627.

Minkler, M. and Wallerstein, N. (2008) *Community-based Participatory Research for Health: From Process to Outcomes*, 2nd edition. San Francisco, CA: Jossey Bass.

Tronto, J.C. (2013) *Caring Democracy. Markets, Equality and Justice.* New York: New York University Press.

1 Community development and hospices

A national UK perspective

Libby Sallnow, Antonia Bunnin and
Heather Richardson

Community and hospices

In the UK, the notions of hospice and community are closely intertwined at conceptual, strategic and operational levels. Many hospices in this country owe their origins, early funding and initial plans to local people or groups who had a vision to create a new service for people dying in their area and who were prepared to donate time, money and effort to make this vision a reality. Such community support remains vital for the majority of hospices even as they are well established and employ large numbers of professionals to deliver care and manage the business of the organisation. Today, nationally, 74 per cent of funding for independent hospices operating in the UK is raised from charitable rather than statutory sources (Hospice UK, 2014), including a significant proportion from community fundraising. Opportunities for, and numbers of, volunteers working in hospices also continue to grow. It is estimated that the UK hospice volunteer workforce now exceeds 125,000 people (Help the Hospices, 2014), who take on a variety of roles including fundraising, care delivery, retail support, contributions as unpaid professionals and governance (Hoad, 1991; Turner and Payne, 2008; Burbeck et al. 2014). The annual financial value of their contribution has been estimated at £133 million in return for an investment of £16.7 million (Gaskin, 2003). The contribution of volunteers is recognised as extending beyond pure financial gains, however, and the impacts on patients and families (Herbst-Damm and Kulik 2005; Block et al., 2010; Candy et al., 2014), on the volunteers themselves (Addington-Hall and Karlsen, 2005; Harris and Thoresen, 2006; Li, 2007) and on broader issues such as social ties and support (McKinnon, 2002) have been widely documented.

This vital relationship between hospices and communities is recognised by the hospice sector. The national umbrella organisation for hospice care – Hospice UK (formerly Help the Hospices) has placed an emphasis on the relationship that hospices have with the communities they serve by highlighting it in its definition of hospice care as 'community engaged palliative and end of life care in all settings for patients, families and carers'

(Help the Hospices, 2012a). This was intended as a means of differentiating hospice care from other forms of palliative and end of life care. Most hospices have put a variety of structures and processes in place to connect the organisation to local people and community groups – including volunteer coordinators and community fundraisers.

Volunteering and hospices

Volunteering, seen as one of the main conduits of connection between hospices and their local communities, has recently come under closer scrutiny with the recognition that the wider impacts of volunteering, besides the financial gains, may be worth investigation (Leadbeater and Garber, 2010). Traditional models of volunteering within hospices focus on recruiting volunteers to fulfil roles required by the hospice, to support them in their service delivery. Differing models from around the world (see Kumar, 2007; and Jack et al., 2011) have prompted many to re-evaluate their current models of volunteer 'management' and to ask whether this resource could be managed differently, to provide benefits beyond the hospice, to the wider community. In so doing, hospices move towards a community development approach.

Sallnow (2010) conducted a systematic review of the literature relating to volunteering in palliative care internationally and developed a conceptual model regarding how volunteering could be understood (Figure 1.1). The literature demonstrated that there are a range of impacts beyond the financial, including wider societal implications. It also demonstrated that key factors in determining what impacts are realised are the motivations and experiences of the local people volunteering and type of management style that governs it. A style that focuses on power sharing and respecting the volunteer as presenting a unique contribution from the local community (an empowering model of management) would be more able to realise these loftier aims of social change, whereas a more restraining model, where the hospice sets the agenda and volunteers arrive to fit predetermined slots, will be less able.

The Commission into the Future of Hospice Care confirmed a need to develop new approaches to volunteering, including models of hospice-owned but volunteer-led services (Help the Hospices, 2012b).

This reappraisal of the role of volunteers within hospice care can be seen to be part of a wider, national refocusing on the relationship people as citizens, rather than patients, have with their statutory, voluntary and other organisations. Involving local people in the decisions that affect them has been included in government papers (Cabinet Office, 2009, 2010; Department of Health, 2011), grass-roots community projects (Social Action for Health, 2012) and research (Oliver et al., 2007) and the impact this can have in health and social care has not gone unnoticed. The links between social support or social networks and health have been demonstrated

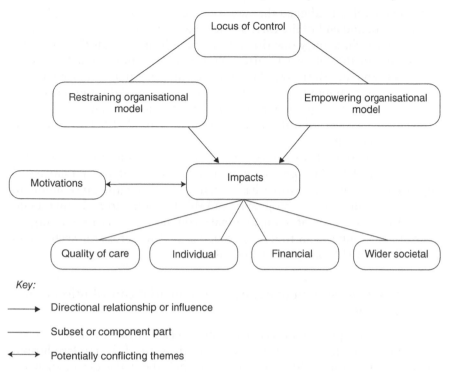

Figure 1.1 A conceptual model of volunteering
Source: Copyright Libby Sallnow, 2010.

(Holt-Lunstad et al. 2010; Reeves et al., 2014) and, increasingly, evidence is suggesting that engaging communities in tackling health issues leads to better results than leaving it solely to professionals (O'Mara-Eves et al., 2013). The findings of reviews such as the Marmot Review (2010) confirm that in order to tackle health inequalities most effectively, local participatory decision making must be enabled. This recognition has led to multi-level policy initiatives in the UK, from the creation of Health and Wellbeing boards being tasked with tackling social isolation (Department of Health, 2012; Buck and Gregory, 2013) to social prescribing (South et al., 2008) to the NHS Alliance releasing its first Community Development Charter (NHS Alliance, 2014), calling on organisations from NHS England to individual commissioners to prioritise the engagement of local people.

Community development and hospices

The role and importance of engaging communities in their own end of life care has been expounded within palliative care since the 1990s and the sector is now looking beyond models of volunteering to radically different means of engagement. Kellehear (1999, 2005; Karapliaglou and Kellehear,

2014) first explicitly aligned the two seemingly contradictory disciplines of public health and end of life care. Services have then taken this 'new' public health approach, namely one that focuses on a health promoting approach as outlined in the Ottawa Charter (WHO, 1986), and applied the same principles of building healthy public policy, creating supportive environments, strengthening community action, developing personal skills and reorienting health services to contemporary end of life care. Examples of such applications exist around the world (Sallnow et al., 2012; Horsfall et al., 2012; McLoughlin, 2013).

Later chapters in this book confirm an increasing interest in new public health in the UK. The predominant interpretation of the public health approach across its four nations has been through 'strengthening community action', or community development, and this has come to be known under the collective heading of 'compassionate communities'. A recent surge in interest and commitment to this approach is evident across the sector (Paul and Sallnow, 2013; Barry and Patel, 2013).

Compassionate communities and their potential contribution to the hospice sector

Although the hospice sector has made unparalleled advances in the care and support of the dying and their families since the start of the modern hospice movement in the late 1960s, questions remain about the extent to which hospices are delivering on their original goal and purpose, and to what extent those original goals are relevant for the different context and environment we find ourselves in today.

The challenges of the twenty-first century are placing new and heavier demands on already stretched health and social care services. A report written by Calanzani et al. (2013) describes a future in which there will be increasing numbers of people who live for extended periods with chronic and life-threatening conditions, many living alone with high levels of disability. The epidemiological transition means we are seeing chronic conditions such as heart disease, cancer and dementia with long trajectories rather than acute forms of infective illnesses with relatively shorter durations. The burden this places on health and social care services is significant, as they were predicated on an acute model of illness. Another corollary of our ageing population is the emergence of social isolation as a major public health concern (Cattan et al., 2005). The rise of single-person households and housebound individuals at the end of life means this is an urgent concern for the field.

The hospice sector has faced criticism over its poor record of access by people from minority ethnic groups (Coupland et al., 2011), those from lesbian, gay, bisexual and transgender (LGBT) communities (Harding et al., 2012), from those with conditions other than cancer or of older people (Ahmed et al., 2004), and low social economic class (Kessler et al., 2005).

Indeed, hospice care has been labelled 'deluxe dying for the few' (Douglas, 1992). Sustained efforts to tackle these issues have led to important changes, for example work by St Joseph's Hospice in East London to increase access for people from minority ethnic groups in the area (Richardson, 2012), but the sector acknowledges that there remains more to be done (Help the Hospices, 2013).

Hospices have also been subject to the critique that they have contributed, albeit unwittingly, to the disempowerment of communities and individuals in relation to end of life care. By professionalising the business of dying, families and communities are pushed to the peripheries as the professionals are viewed as the only ones who can support someone who is dying. Coupled with this is the concern regarding the medicalisation of palliative care, with critics suggesting that medical or psychological symptom management is prioritised at the expense of social issues. Kellehear (1999) writes convincingly of the gap that is emerging in a model of care that fails to acknowledge the social experience of dying and loss and which is concerned almost entirely with the management of physical symptoms. This tension extends beyond care of the dying person to those who face loss. Nyatanga (2014) warns the palliative care world of pathologising grief and seeking to manage it, rather than seeing it as a natural process with inevitable chaos. This, combined with the fear local communities may have about their role and what they are allowed to do when someone is dying, means communities step back and ask for professional support, even though they may have been fulfilling a particular role for a person for many years. Recently, there has been increasing realisation that these community roles and strengths need to be supported and that professionals should endeavour to fit into the gaps around them. This requires a different approach, to look at strengths and assets, rather than just needs. The NHS Alliance suggests 'looking at what is strong and not wrong' (NHS Alliance, 2014).

Finally, the current fiscal climate means hospices and other voluntary organisations are struggling to provide a comprehensive service with current funding streams. With the predicted increases in deaths year on year, the current models of inpatient, specialist palliative care will not be able to meet these demands and, as discussed above, are not the most appropriate models of care to be rolled out. More collaborative and community-focused care will be required, building on the strengths of local communities and working in partnership with community members, other health and social care providers and the hospice. This will not only deliver more appropriate and sustainable care but care that in the long run is more financially viable.

Models of compassionate communities in end of life care

The literature has begun to offer some examples of compassionate communities in end of life care in England and Scotland. Barry and Patel (2013) catalogued approaches under the compassionate communities heading and describe 28 case studies across England. The case studies described in this book provide further detail of the work that has developed. What is clear is that there is mixed understanding about what a community development approach or a compassionate community comprises and how this compares to an awareness-raising initiative or a traditional volunteer service. In order to support understanding of this subtle difference, Sallnow and Paul (2014) built on learning in other sectors, to develop a spectrum of engagement in end of life care (Figure 1.2).

The spectrum extends from informing, to consulting, co-production, collaboration and finally to empowerment. As each stage is reached, the levels of power sharing between the organisation and the community increase until communities take ownership of aspects of care and support. It is this power sharing and participation that distinguishes compassionate community approaches from more traditional models of volunteer use, awareness-raising or public education.

Numerous different models of public health approaches to end of life care have developed, in part due to the diversity of need. Some start at the level of the carer and family and support them individually, helping them to mobilise their own networks, whilst some support the community to develop the capacity to support those living among them. Others focus more on interacting with community organisations such as schools, religious institutions and local businesses to enable messages about healthy dying and societal support for those in need. Still others focus on policy-level initiatives, to create the environment and tools for change, or on participative public education events to support death awareness and literacy. Environmental change has been used by some to transform settings to make them more conducive to supporting those in need and others simply recognise and capture naturally occurring compassionate communities work that can exist within communities and support and develop these efforts.

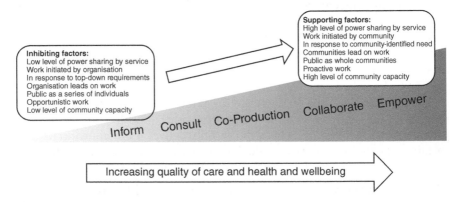

Figure 1.2 A spectrum of engagement in end of life care: developing community capacity

Source: Sallnow and Paul (2014), reproduced with permission from Taylor and Francis.

Challenges facing hospices interested in community development

Although the new public health approach to end of life care is often presented as a panacea for the hospice sector's ills, there remain numerous and substantial difficulties in achieving widespread gains through this work. Health promotion and community development are notoriously difficult fields in which to understand processes of change, to demonstrate impacts and outcomes, and to authentically engage with communities. Consideration of these important issues to community development in end of life care is no exception. This next section outlines some of the major issues and challenges facing the hospice sector if it is to realise the anticipated potential of these approaches.

One issue is that thus far there has been relatively limited theoretical understanding of community development within the sector. Although the number of initiatives is growing and admirable, inspiration to date has been drawn from a relatively narrow range of sources, and based on the work of a few key authors (for example Kellehear, 1999; Kumar, 2007; Leadbeater and Garber, 2010), and practice examples. Often change has been driven by one or two leaders within a hospice but because the ideas are not yet widely understood across the sector, these leaders have had to expend a great deal of energy on driving and embedding *local* change which is often relatively *small scale* in terms of numbers/communities engaged with, and thus in terms of (likely) impact. As the number of community development and compassionate communities initiatives grows, a key challenge is to share ongoing learning across the sector, and especially to explore together how these approaches can be effectively scaled.

There has also been a tendency for hospices to draw on examples from within end of life care, but not yet to utilise a wider range of theoretical models and approaches such as Asset-Based Community Development (ABCD), Appreciative Inquiry, peer research, participatory research and planning methodologies, logic models or theories of change, nor to draw on expertise in community development from outside the sector, with a few notable exceptions where hospices have begun to establish relationships with community development and public health experts.

A challenge the hospice sector now faces is to collectively develop an increasingly sophisticated understanding of community development – including the range of approaches and techniques available, when and how best to deploy them, and what type of impacts can be expected – through continuing to share experiences and learning, and through drawing on expertise from outside the sector.

Tackling the challenges

Moving beyond a professional rhetoric

The voices, interests and lived experiences of people with end of life care needs (patients, families, bereaved people and members of local communities) are currently still relatively unheard within most hospice community development work. The work has been initiated and driven by hospice professionals and academics, and in many cases has been at the early stages of the engagement spectrum, yet there is growing interest in how to shift towards the higher levels of the spectrum, towards genuine co-production, collaboration and empowerment of people – both those currently with end of life care needs, and members of local communities. (This was a central topic of debate at a Compassionate Communities Practitioners Day held by Weston Hospicecare in association with Hospice UK in September 2014.) If hospices can widen staff skills, draw on expertise from outside the sector and increase use of techniques such as asset-based, participatory and Appreciate Inquiry approaches within their community development work, these steps should help to ensure greater participant/user voice, reduce professional dominance and achieve the desired shift.

Establishing effective models of community development

There is limited understanding – even amongst those working in hospice community development – of the strengths and weaknesses of different models, and the connections between different approaches/processes and intended outcomes. Historically, one of the great strengths of the sector has been the ability of hospices – operating mainly as independent charities rather than part of the state – to experiment; initiating and developing new local services relatively quickly and without huge bureaucracy. This is illustrated in the way that a few visionary and energetic leaders have been able to introduce and drive community development initiatives in their hospices and local communities. The result has been the creation of different practice models, according to differing local needs, interests, context and skills. However, the way community development has evolved to date within the hospice sector – and the fact that many projects are still at an early stage – means there have been only limited attempts to create a shared theory of change, set of conceptual models or shared evaluative frameworks. The time is now right for hospices to work together to look more deeply at what works and why.

The aims of hospice community development initiatives tend to be high level, strategic and aspirational – sometimes incorporated in some way into a hospice's new strategic vision or plan. But there is currently no set of established processes or methodology for any given hospice to use to then translate these into a more detailed set of objectives, and from there into well-informed decisions about the best approaches and techniques to deploy, the actions required to achieve those objectives, and an articulation of *how* those actions will achieve the objectives.

Hospices have relatively limited experience to date of evaluating their community development work, but will need to develop a much better understanding of the links between processes and outcomes, if they are to start to introduce and learn from such evaluations. These concerns are not unique to hospice community development; there is active interest within other areas of hospice and palliative care – especially clinical care – about how best to implement outcome measures, strengthen the role of evaluation and benchmarking, and use the findings to shape ongoing improvements. New techniques such as the Medical Research Council (MRC) complex intervention framework (Anderson, 2008) and techniques utilised in health promotion and community development may also prove useful.

The drive for better understanding of the links between processes and outcomes in community development is not unproblematic; there are tensions and trade-offs that hospices face between having very clearly defined aims, objectives and actions at the outset of any community development initiative, or having looser aims and a more iterative approach to deciding objectives and actions – less tied to goals, metrics and performance indicators. The former risks being overly prescriptive, creating risk-aversion and limiting scope for creativity, learning and adaptation, especially in light of initial feedback and insights gained from people using services and/or local communities. The latter fits more closely with the ethos of responsive and empowering community development, as well as with the model of the inspirational leader who creates enthusiasm and energy for the idea of 'trying something new'. But it also risks giving rise to situations where hospices are unable to articulate 'what success looks like', nor to measure how effective (or, indeed, cost-effective) their community development work has been; or else just focus on inputs/activities (what they have done) rather than on outcomes and impact (what difference they have made).

'Managing'risk appropriately

The issues of how to understand and manage risk in relation to community development work present further challenges for hospices. This was a matter of considerable interest at the Compassionate Communities Practitioners Day in September 2014 referred to above, especially regarding how hospices work with members of local communities who are engaged to support others who are unwell or dying. The question was asked: Where do you draw the line between being a volunteer and a friend? As hospices move away from traditional models of recruiting, training and then monitoring volunteers, towards approaches focused on strengthening capacity of people in a local community to support others, including through informal social networks, they are finding that these new approaches do not always sit easily with their existing policies and procedures, organisational culture and expectations, and established models of governance.

Establishing strategic coherence

Any hospice undertaking community development work faces the challenge of ensuring strategic coherence with the rest of the hospice's work. Some have been accused of 'mission drift' – an issue of much discussion at the Help the Hospices Conference in 2012, which focused on community engagement and hospice care. How should hospices decide what is the 'right' balance (and allocation of resource) between providing palliative care to people with a terminal diagnosis or at very end of life, and their public health and community development work which may include developing 'upstream' interventions; raising awareness about dying, loss and grief; overcoming fears and taboos about death and hospices; and building trust and relationships with specific communities, even prior to such upstream interventions? What are the implications for perceptions of the hospice locally, for their fundraising and their positioning in local partnerships?

If hospices can develop a more sophisticated and evidence-based understanding of the various models and theoretical frameworks available, this would assist hospice leaders to think more clearly with others to reach such decisions about balance and resource allocation, and also help them to explain and justify their community development work.

Being clear about the outcomes required

There are particular challenges involved in any community development initiative intended to build community capacity or social capital, defined by Putnam (1995) as 'social connections and the attendant norms and trust'. Whilst this is easy to include as a high-level aim, measurement of social capital, and of the effectiveness of actions intended to increase it, is notoriously difficult. Hospices that state an intention to build social capital or community capacity need to ask a further set of questions: *Why* build social capital – is this an end in itself or as a means to a specific end? (The former answer may risk concerns about mission drift or straying beyond charitable objects.) Amongst *whom* – which parts of the community? *What kinds* of social capital are we seeking to build (bonding or bridging; formal or informal, etc.)? *How* will we do this? And how will we tell whether we have succeeded; how will we *measure and evaluate* success?

These issues are not easy to address, but the potential benefits are significant. Conversely, a failure to ask themselves questions such as those set out above, coupled with weak articulation of the connections between process and outcomes and a lack of evaluation, will heighten the risk that hospices may (intentionally or not) end up paying lip service to community development – introducing changes with superficial or limited effect, and without the sustained energy and conscious ceding of power and authority necessary for genuine co-production, collaboration and empowerment of individuals and local communities. It also increases the risk of romanticisation, where any initiative labelled community development is deemed inherently laudable, without further critical analysis.

Final thoughts

This chapter provides an overview of the potential contribution and some of the challenges for hospices interested in community development. The authors bring a range of experiences in this issue – of local development, evaluation and national support of hospice efforts related to a public health approach to death, dying and loss. We hope that it will serve as helpful context to the case studies provided in other parts of the book that describe the work of local hospices to establish compassionate communities.

One of our reflections on completion of this chapter is that much effort is still required on the part of hospices and many other stakeholders to make the aspiration of hospices as effective public health agents, one that can be achieved. Our labouring of the challenges facing hospices and how they can be overcome reflects our belief that if hospices address these challenges successfully they could have significant impact in redressing many of the gaps in provision that have led them to look at alternative means of providing care in the future.

In terms of the way forward we urge consideration of the following. First, that hospices interested in this approach continue to build relationships with each other, and also with organisations beyond the sector. We hope that they will look for partnerships with public health colleagues, with academic centres, with community development organisations or others with expertise in this area. We hope also that they will engage carefully and closely with community leaders and other individuals of influence who can influence and support local change. We are keen that academic centres give consideration to models of change and evaluation that focus on outcomes most appropriate to this work. We urge funders to consider ongoing support in this area – such efforts and their evaluation require sustained input if they are to be successful ultimately. Most importantly we urge all to continue to think critically about what role hospices play in this agenda in the future and how they are best positioned to achieve it.

References

Addington-Hall, J.M. and Karlsen, S. (2005) A national survey of health professionals and volunteers working in voluntary hospices in the UK. II. Staff and volunteers' experiences of working in hospices. *Palliative Medicine* 19(1): 49–57.

Ahmed, N., Bestall, J.E., Ahmedzai, S., Payne, S.A., Clark, D. and Noble, B. (2004) Systematic review of the problems and issues of accessing specialist palliative care by patients, carers and health and social care professionals. *Palliative Medicine* 18(6): 525–542.

Anderson, R. (2008) New MRC guidance on evaluating complex interventions. *BMJ* 2008;337:a1937.

Barry, V. and Patel, M. (2013) *An Overview of Compassionate Communities in England*. London: Murray Hall Community Trust; National Council for Palliative Care Dying Matters.

Block, E., Casarett, D.J., Spence, C., Gozalo, P., Connor, S.R. and Teno, J.M. (2010) Got volunteers? Association of hospice use of volunteers with bereaved family members' overall rating of the quality of end-of-life care. *Journal of Pain and Symptom Management* 39(3): 502–506.

Buck, G., and Gregory, S. (2013) *Improving the Public's Health. A Resource for Local Authorities.* London: The King's Fund.

Burbeck, R., Low, J., Sampson, E., Bravery, R., Hill, M., Morris, S., et al. (2014) Volunteers in specialist palliative care: a survey of adult services in the United Kingdom. *Palliative Medicine* 17(5): 568–574.

Cabinet Office. (2009) *Real Help for Communities: Volunteers, Charities and Social Enterprises.* London: Cabinet Office.

Cabinet Office. (2010) *Building the Big Society.* London: Cabinet Office.

Calanzani, N., Higginson, I.J. and Gomes, B. (2013) Current and future needs for hospice care: an evidence-based report. A Report for the Commission into the Future of Hospice Care. London: Help the Hospices.

Candy, B., France, R., Low, J. and Sampson, L. (2014) Does involving volunteers in the provision of palliative care make a difference to patient and family wellbeing? A systematic review of quantitative and qualitative evidence. *International Journal of Nursing Studies.* Aug 23. pii: S0020-7489(14)00210-7. doi: 10.1016/j.ijnurstu.2014.08.007.

Cattan, M., White, M., Bond, J. and Learmouth, A. (2005) Preventing social isolation and loneliness among older people: a systematic review of health promotion interventions. *Ageing and Society* 25: 41–67.

Coupland, V., Madden, P., Jack, R.H., Moller, H. and Davies, E.A. (2011) Does place of death from cancer vary between ethnic groups in South East England? *Palliative Medicine* 25(4): 314–322.

Department of Health. (2011) *Social Action for Health and Wellbeing: Building Cooperative Communities: Department of Health Strategic Vision for volunteering.* London: Stationery Office.

Department of Health. (2012) *Health and Social Care Act.* London: Stationery Office.

Douglas, C. (1992) For all the saints. *BMJ* 304: 579.

Gaskin, K. (2003) *The Economics of Hospice Volunteering.* London: Help the Hospices.

Harding, R., Epiphaniou, E. and Chidgey-Clark, J. (2012) Needs, experiences, and preferences of sexual minorities for end-of-life care and palliative care: a systematic review. *Palliative Medicine* 15(5): 602–611.

Harris, A.H. and Thoresen, C.E. (2006) Volunteer befriending as an intervention for depression: implications for bereavement care. *Bereavement Care* 25(2): 27–30.

Help the Hospices. (2012a) *Strategic Plan 2012–2016.* London: Help the Hospices.

Help the Hospices. (2012b) Volunteers: vital to the future of hospice care. A Report for the Commission into the Future of Hospice Care. London: Help the Hospices.

Help the Hospices. (2013) Future ambitions for hospice care: our mission and our opportunity. The Report of the Commission into the Future of Hospice Care. London: Help the Hospices.

Help the Hospices. (2014) New exhibition showcases rich legacy of hospice volunteering. Press Release, February. http://www.hospiceuk.org/media-centre/press-releases/details/2014/02/27/new-exhibition-showcases-rich-legacy-of-hospice-volunteering

Herbst-Damm, K.L. and Kulik, J.A. (2005) Volunteer support, marital status, and the survival times of terminally ill patients. *Health Psychology* 24(2): 225–229.

Hoad, P. (1991) Volunteers in the independent hospice movement. *Sociology of Health and Illness* 13(2): 231–248.

Holt-Lunstad, J., Smith, T.B. and Layton, J.B. (2010) Social relationships and mortality risk: a meta-analytic review. *PLoS Medicine* 7(7) e1000316.

Horsfall, D., Noonan, K. and Leonard, R. (2012) Bringing our dying home: how caring for someone at the end of life builds social capital and develops compassionate communities. *Health Sociology Review* 21(4): 373–382.

Hospice UK. (2014) *Hospice Accounts: Analysis of the Accounts of UK Independent Voluntary Hospices for the Year Ended 31 March 2013*. London: Hospice UK.

Jack, B., Kirton, J., Birakurataki, J. and Merriman, A. (2011) 'A bridge to the hospice': the impact of a Community Volunteer Programme in Uganda. *Palliative Medicine* 25(7): 706–715.

Karapliaglou, A. and Kellehear, A. (2014) *Public Health Approaches to End of Life Care. A Toolkit*. London: National Council for Palliative Care, Public Health England and Middlesex University.

Kellehear, A. (1999) *Health-promoting Palliative Care*. Melbourne: Oxford University Press.

Kellehear, A. (2005) *Compassionate Cities: Public Health and End-of-Life Care*. London: Routledge.

Kessler, D., Peters, T.J., Lee, L. and Parr, S. (2005) Social class and access to specialist palliative care services. *Palliative Medicine* 19(2): 105–110.

Kumar, S. (2007) Kerala, India: a regional community-based palliative care model. *Journal of Pain and Symptom Management* 33(5): 623–627.

Leadbeater, C. and Garber, J. (2010) *Dying for Change*. London: Demos.

Li, L. (2007) Recovering from spousal bereavement in later life: does volunteer participation play a role? *Journal of Gerontology* 62B(4): S257–S266.

McKinnon, M. (2002) The participation of volunteers in contemporary palliative care. *Australian Journal of Advanced Nursing* 19(4): 38–44.

McLoughlin, K. (2013) *Compassionate Communities Evaluation Report*. Limerick: Milford Care Centre.

Marmot Review. (2010) *Fair Society Healthy Lives*. London: Marmot Review.

NHS Alliance. (2014) *A Charter for Community Development in Health*. London: NHS Alliance.

Nyatanga, B. (2014) A century of pathologising grief and bereavement. *International Journal of Palliative Care Nursing* 20(7): 315–315.

O'Mara-Eves, A., Brunton, G., McDaid, D., Kavanagh, J., Jamal, F., Matosevic, T., et al. (2013) Community engagement to reduce inequalities in health: a systematic review, meta-analysis and economic analysis. *Public Health Research* 1(4): 1–141.

Oliver, S.R., Ress, R.W., Clarke-Jones, L., Milne, R., Oakley, A.R., Gabbay, J., et al. (2007) A multidimensional conceptual framework for analysing public involvement in health services research. *Health Expectations* 11: 72–84.

Paul, S. and Sallnow, L. (2013) Public health approaches to end of life care in the UK: an online survey of palliative care services. *BMJ: Supportive and Palliative Care* 3: 196–199.

Putnam, R.D. (1995) Bowling alone: America's declining social capital. *Journal of Democracy* 6: 65–78.

Reeves, D., Blickem. C., Vassilev, I., Brooks, H., Kennedy, A., Richardson, G. and Rogers, A. (2014) The contribution of social networks to the health and self-management of patients with long-term conditions: a longitudinal study. *PLoS Medicine* 9(6): e98340.

Richardson, H. (2012) A public health approach to palliative care in East London – early developments, challenges and plans for the future. In: Sallnow, L., Kumar, S. and Kellehear, A. (eds) *International Perspectives on Public Health and Palliative Care*. Abingdon: Routledge.

Sallnow, L. (2010) Conceptualisation of volunteering in palliative care: a narrative synthesis of the literature. Master's thesis, Kings College London.

Sallnow, L. and Paul, S. (2014) Understanding community engagement in end-of-life care: developing conceptual clarity. *Critical Public Health* doi: 10.1080/09581596.2014.909582

Sallnow, L., Kumar, S. and Kellehear, A. (eds) (2012) *International Perspectives on Public Health and Palliative Care*. Abingdon: Routledge.

Social Action for Health. (2012) *Annual Report*. London: Social Action for Health.

South, J., Higgins, T.J., Woodall, J. and White, S.M. (2008) Can social prescribing provide the missing link? *Primary Health Care Research & Development* 9: 310–318.

Turner. M. and Payne, S. (2008) Uncovering the hidden volunteers in palliative care: a survey of hospice trustees in the United Kingdom. *Palliative Medicine* 22(8): 973–974.

World Health Organisation (WHO). (1986) Ottawa Charter for Health Promotion. Ottawa: WHO.

2 Developing community support networks at the end of life in Weston-super-Mare, UK

Julian Abel and Ditch Townsend

Weston-super-Mare is a small town in the south west of England. Weston Hospicecare provides specialist palliative care for the town and surrounding villages, covering a total population of approximately 150,000 people. The hospice has a 10-bed inpatient unit, a specialist palliative care community team providing specialist support for people in their homes and a day centre. Over the last five years, in addition to the usual specialist palliative care approach of the physical, social, psychological and spiritual, the hospice as an organisation has developed increasing interest and expertise in public health approaches to end of life care. This has mainly focused on developing and enhancing naturally occurring supportive networks that surround patients and their families. The project described below has been the main focus of our efforts, although we increasingly are becoming involved in a variety of other related initiatives. Dr Abel is the Medical Director at the hospice and spends half of his time working there. The other half is as a palliative care consultant at Weston Area Health Trust, a small district general hospital. Ditch Townsend is employed as the compassionate community network coordinator. His background is in international community development, particularly in Asia. He was employed specifically for the project by the hospice.

National context

In 2006, the then Labour government produced a White Paper, *Our Health, Our Care, Our Say : A New Direction for Community Services* (Department of Health, 2006). The foundation of this paper was a public consultation, Your Health, Your Care, Your Say. One of the areas highlighted by the public was that although more than 50 per cent of people would choose to die at home, only 20 per cent actually did so. At the time, more than half of all deaths in England were in hospital. The White Paper set out the formation of a national end of life network. In 2008 the national *End of Life Care Strategy* (Department of Health, 2008) was published. A central theme of this document was that people should be asked about where they would choose to die; these wishes should be recorded for the broader health and social care community to see; the wishes should be respected and that coordinated care should be given to allow someone to die in their place of choice. The strategy resulted in a nationwide effort to improve end of life services and, as a consequence, there has been a year on year reduction in percentage hospital death rate. By 2014, this had fallen to below 50 per cent (Network, 2014a). However, the percentage home death rate has only risen by 2 percentage points in that time, with the major contributor to this increase being an increase in the home death rate for cancer. By and large, the palliative care community have been the major instigators of improvements in end of life care and historically the largest proportion of their patients have been those with a diagnosis of cancer.

The reasons for the only very modest improvements in home death rate are complex. Part of the problem has been the reluctance of health care professionals to identify those people in the last months or years of life and have a conversation with them about end of life planning. This is particularly the case for non cancer terminal illnesses where prediction of prognosis may be difficult. People can live for many years with severe, end-stage illness and at the same time others may die as a result of a sudden deterioration. The natural history of incurable cancer tends to have a more predictable course. It is then hard to be able to coordinate a home death with appropriate care if someone has not made the choice to die at home before the final days of their illness. Preparing the family for the care and nursing that is needed requires careful consideration, addressing their worries and concerns, and ensuring that appropriate medication is available in the home. Even when advance care planning has been completed, arranging care services at home can be complicated. Once these services are in place, they are not universally popular with patients and carers, as they might involve many different professional carers entering the house each week. Often, the time of arrival of the care staff is fitted into their busy schedule and does not necessarily meet the needs or the timing for their patients. Care given is task-oriented and time-limited. It is not unusual for patients and carers to be reluctant to accept care, and even when care has been accepted, it may be turned away for the same reasons.

The natural focus on professional care, from the perspective of health and social care professionals, however, does not necessarily have the same degree of focus for patients and families. Burns et al. (2013) showed that the bulk of care, including hands-on care, is given by extended family members (non first degree relatives) and friends.

The problems of professional care have been further complicated in recent years by the financial crisis that started in 2008. Spiralling health costs, with increased usage of health services in all settings, with a limited supply of money have meant that the availability of care packages is decreasing. There has been significant reduction in social care funding. At the same time, the increased use of advance care planning, where people are choosing to die at home rather than in public institutions, has placed further stress on the system. In some localities, gains made in allowing people to die in their usual place of residence have slowed down and even decreased (Network, 2014b).

The increasing professionalisation of dying and death, since the formation of the hospice movement and formation of palliative care as a speciality, has seen communities develop the expectation that professional services will provide end of life care (Abel et al., 2011). This has resulted in a loss of familiarity of communities of how to care for those people who are dying in the community itself. This is at odds with the increasing desire for people to die at home. Who is going to provide the care?

The role of public health approaches including community development

Community development offers solutions to some of these problems. How can communities themselves increase their ability to care for people at end of life, not just in the final days of life but the final weeks, months and years? How can communities continue to support people through bereavement, whether the death of their loved one is sudden or after a prolonged illness, whether young or old?

Our own project was born out of these considerations, stimulated by the work of Allan Kellehear (2005). Our fundamental consideration was how we could enhance the naturally occurring supportive networks that already surround people at end of life. This was not aimed solely at the final days of illness, but looking to enhance the capacity of networks to care, from diagnosis through to bereavement and beyond. Many people would like to live the final phase of their life surrounded by the people they love, in the environment they are familiar with and have shaped themselves over many years. This is often true wherever people die and, for many, they would want this to be at home. We felt that the hospice was a good starting point to look to enhance community networks, as this was seen already as a part of what we do. We were aware that although community and particularly family support was part of our routine consideration, we often turned to professional services as a first port of call when we felt more care was needed. This could be at the point of crisis, where carers were struggling to cope with someone at home. Our project aimed to start to develop naturally occurring supportive networks at an earlier point in the illness, to try and preserve community resilience for when the care needs, both physical and emotional, became more pressing.

Most importantly for us, we felt that the supporting naturally occurring networks would result in more people living and dying in their communities, surrounded and supported by the people who were closest to them. This felt to us to be the right thing to do, and could enhance a sense of meaning and value for patients, carers and those in the caring network, whether this was through direct patient contact or indirectly by supporting carers. The possible solutions to lack of availability of professional carers and the need to decrease costs were of secondary importance, although we realised that from a commissioning perspective, these could easily be seen as powerful drivers for such a project.

Project development

During our background research, we became aware of a similar project that had been running in Sydney, Australia, for many years. An extensive report (Horsfall et al., 2012) described the benefits of enhancing naturally occurring networks, using a volunteer mentor who had been through the experience of caring for a loved one who died. Because of the many similarities of this project to the one we envisaged, we contacted the authors and initially arranged a Skype conversation with them. This was followed by a visit to Australia to learn in more detail how they set up and ran their project, as well as how they ran the evaluation. This proved to be extremely helpful and, following our visit, we were able to set up a project plan.

Organisational culture change

As we investigated further and thought about community development as an approach, we began to understand that a radical shift in our thinking was needed. During the trip to Australia, we formulated ideas of how we might explain this to our organisation and eventually published an article describing this theoretical basis (Abel et al., 2013). This radical shift would need to be supported at all levels of the organisation, including the Board of Trustees, the senior management team, the clinical teams and the fundraising teams. We had already begun to talk about our plans some while previously and the trustees had kindly permitted us to use an educational support fund for the trip to Australia. Over the ensuing weeks and months, we talked about the practical application of community development in clinical settings, discussed our paper at our local journal club meetings and debated our approach at the senior management team meetings.

The essence of what we were trying to get across was that naturally occurring supportive networks already surround people who have terminal illnesses, to a greater or lesser degree. We needed to actively enhance these networks by supporting patients and carers to mobilise them. This was not so that professional care services were not used, but that there was an active partnership between them and informal networks. Rather than reaching towards professional care as the first answer to care problems, we needed to start enabling informal networks at as early a stage of the illness as possible. What we wanted to do was shift our focus from the professionals to naturally occurring supportive networks as a starting point. This was more of a change of emphasis rather than doing something entirely new.

The discussions we had proved to be quite challenging for many professionals. The implication is that supportive networks can do some of what health and social care professionals do, whether this is physical care or emotional support. This then calls into question the role of the professional carer, which in turn questions their role and their value. Continued discussion, particularly at the multidisciplinary meeting was helpful in addressing some of these concerns, with a refocus on how we consider physical and social caring networks. Some people understood this better than others and we found that, for example, our complementary therapy team leader was able to apply principles in a practical way, generating clear narratives of change. These helped clinicians understand how the principles of community development work in practice.

Having begun to embed our ideas, our fundraising department applied successfully for a Big Lottery grant, part of the National Lottery in England aimed at supporting community projects. We then appointed our project coordinator, who had significant experience in community development, particularly using participatory methodology, in a wide variety of international settings.

A model for supporting end of life community networks

Our model involved:

a   Coordinator employment
b   Volunteer, ex-carer, community companion development
c   Clinical team referral
d   Carer support
e   Network development
f   Bereavement support.

Coordinator employment

We looked for someone who had experience of project management, community development, and had some familiarity with end of life care. The community development and project management aspects were of primary importance to us, as we wanted someone who would be able to set up an appropriate programme, develop it and be able to fulfil the reporting requirements of the funding body. Participatory development seeks to engage the participants, i.e. those people who would benefit from a project, in determining how the project should be configured and run. This can be quite challenging for professionals, as it relies on the expertise and knowledge of the participants rather than the professionals. In our context, the professionals should be enablers of participants rather than determining how the project is to be run.

Volunteer, ex-carer, community companion development

The central part of our project revolved around the benefits of having a community companion. With the community companion having been through the experience of caring for someone, they were expected to have knowledge and insight of how to manage. The suitability of the person in fulfilling this role would be partly determined (on both sides) during the training period. Shared experience is a way of embedding trust so recognition of the difficulties of coping with being a main carer is an important way of building relationships. The community companion could therefore be of benefit by listening to the carer and recognising their experiences having had similar ones themselves. They could be in a position to offer solutions to problems or to allow difficult experiences to be viewed as being normal in the context of caring for a loved one with a terminal illness.

The coordinator was responsible for setting up a steering group, made up from a mixture of hospice professionals and carers, who would oversee the project. He enrolled volunteers and designed the training programme under their guidance. He sought volunteers from people who were already known to the hospice, approaching groups of carers who were already involved with the hospice in a variety of ways. This was through our carers group (aimed at providing peer support for people already involved in caring for a loved one with a terminal illness), our buddies group (aimed at peer support for bereaved people who have been through the carers group) and another service of companion sitters (volunteers who spend time with patients as a source of short respite for carers or to sit with people who have limited non-professional care). Given that our programme was new and novel to the hospice, we wanted to feel our way initially with people who were already familiar to us.

The training was based on the programme from Sydney but adapted to the needs of our project including a degree of corporate wariness. The training structure was defined by the committee and consisted of:

- The work of a hospice
- Signposting
- End of life
- Supervision and self-care
- Communication
- Appropriate activities including Facilitation, Participation, Social network mapping
- Bereavement
- Boundaries.

Clinical team referral

The weekly multidisciplinary meeting at the hospice plays a central role for review of patient care. It offers the opportunity to discuss different initiatives in the hospice. We have found this educational aspect is a good environment to influence the culture of clinical teams. Prior to the project starting, over a period of about one year, we had been discussing the role of enhancing naturally occurring supportive community networks. We considered when this would be appropriate and how we could support carers in developing their own networks. These types of discussions meant that by the time the project was up and running, the clinical teams were already familiar with the type of scenarios where the use of a community companion might prove to be beneficial. Significantly, our project coordinator attended the multidisciplinary meeting. Discussion about referrals could then take place at the meeting. The specialist palliative care community nurse, based on the outcome of the meeting, could then go back to the carer to see if they wanted to have a community companion.

Initially, there was some uncertainty about how to do this. It was felt that the patient needed to give consent for the referral. However, the main beneficiary of our project was the carer. Of course, this would benefit the patient but not always directly. Given that support for the carer would not necessarily involve the patient in a direct way, we agreed that the person to ask would actually be the carer.

Emotional support

Our expectation was that the community companion would build a relationship with the carer. We hoped that having someone who had experience of being a carer for a dying person themselves would give the carer a sense of confidence in the community companion. Building a relationship would then allow the development of the two main functions of the community companion. First this was a listening ear, offering emotional support to the carer, checking on their welfare. Recognition of a shared experience of being a carer is a helpful way of normalising that experience, not seeing it as something wrong or something that is not allowed.

Network development

Caring at the end of life was likened more to a marathon than a sprint and therefore help from a variety of sources could make a big difference. The second role of the community companion was therefore to support carers to develop their own informal networks.

In their paper on naturally occurring supportive networks at end of life, Leonard et al. (2013) describe inner and outer networks. The inner networks are those that have close contact between network participants, with strong relationships, and these are the people who most often will have contact with the patient. The outer network relates more to the less strong bonds, with people being involved in a variety of supportive ways not directly related to patient care. Both of these networks are fundamentally important and have a part to play in increasing the resilience of a patient's main informal carers.

For the health professional it is perhaps easier to understand and relate to the inner network. The tasks involved relate to more traditional care needs, washing, dressing, etc. Of course, the reality of the experience is much broader than this. It encompasses the less tangible aspects of community, including the value of spending time with family and friends, with listening and supporting in a variety of ways.

The outer network also functions in this way but perhaps the focus is more on the carer. As we described in the 'Circles of Care' paper (Abel et al., 2013), the outer network consists of people not as close as those in the inner network but who are not strangers to the family. This includes less close family members, friends and neighbours who may respond to requests for help. The type of tasks that the outer network can do may relate to the sometimes mundane practicalities of living including activities outside the home (e.g. bringing meals, shopping, mowing the lawn, walking the dog). Whilst these tasks in themselves may not be time-consuming or difficult, together they add up to what can be an untenable stress when combined with being a main carer. Tasks can be taken up by different people in the outer network. These may be quite achievable in terms of time and effort in a normally busy life. The overall impact of doing this can be significant, providing support for the carer for what can be a marathon rather than a sprint, creating capacity and space for the carer to attend to what is most needed. This can save carer exhaustion. It can enhance meaning by demonstrating in a real way the community's value for the person with terminal illness.

Large networks require more coordination. If all the coordination falls to the primary carer, organising the network is a further workload, so ideally the carer will have help with the coordination perhaps from someone in the inner network or perhaps from a community-oriented service.

Health and social care professionals tend to think about care being related to need. However, our project incorporates need but is not limited to it. Having someone mow the lawn may not necessarily fit into the needs category. Nevertheless, having someone come round and do this as an act of kindness can have a profound impact, both on the person who mows the lawn and on the grateful recipients of care and help.

The role of the supportive community, including inner and outer networks, is therefore more than just meeting needs. It is about making carers and patients feel like they are supported by kind people who surround them. This is a counterbalance to the feelings of isolation, loss, sense of burden and loss of a sense of value that people experience, whether they are a patient or a carer. Supportive networks symbolise the opposite of this. The symbolic value of acts of kindness when people can feel as though they do not merit it can magnify the impact many times.

At the start of our project, following on from the example of the Australian project, the role of the community companion did not include helping out directly with caring or assisting tasks. Rather, the community companion would try to enable the carer to examine their own network and look to see who could be more effectively involved. The hope was that the carer would feel strong enough to say yes to help when people offered it, and could also ask people for help.

Bereavement support

A common experience for people who are bereaved is that when their loved one dies, particularly after the funeral, they can feel lonely and isolated. This is naturally part of bereavement but caring networks tend to subside after someone has died. We therefore encouraged the community companions to help the carer maintain family and friend support after the death. The community companion would remain as a support up until the one-year anniversary of the death.

Outcomes

We conducted an evaluation 18 months into our project. We supported 39 carers; 29 became bereaved. The average caring period was six and a half months.

Coordinator employment

We employed a former health development manager, with experience of both participatory and traditional community development, who had also supported peer-based care for people in Asia marginalised with AIDS and leprosy.

Volunteer, ex-carer, community companion development

By mid-project, we appeared on track with 17 community companions having completed training or on their way to doing so. But only 6 were confident enough to ever begin practice, and 2 of these had withdrawn. We had started recruitment 'close to home' as planned – indeed all active community companions came from our earliest in-house personal approaches.

Clinical team referral

The multidisciplinary team meeting proved useful for dissecting and establishing the benefits of referral in certain cases, and re-emphasising its benefits in general (when referrals sometimes petered out). But referrals tended to happen from clinical teams outside its confines, although we sometimes simply didn't have enough community companions to help.

Referrals to the community companion service were mostly from the multidisciplinary meeting, with a lesser number coming from informal contacts between teams. We realised if the referrals were made late in the patient's illness, then the opportunity for establishing relationships, giving emotional support and network development became limited. We therefore planned to have an opt-out of referral for community companion support.

There sometimes appeared to be confusion about whether clinical team members were offering a community companion to a carer (which was often refused) or follow-up support to a carer (which was often accepted).

Emotional support and network development

The majority of the contact between our community companions and carers proved to be emotional support. Community companions talked explicitly of their being drawn to the 'pastoral' (non-religious) element of the initiative. As one noted during the evaluation, 'I was a "stranger" prepared to listen without upset or judgement.' It became clear that network development is an incremental, organic process. A common theme for carers is that when their loved one is diagnosed, family, friends and neighbours express sorrow at the news and offer support. Mostly, carers will say no, thinking that they are managing at the moment and they do not want to be a burden. After people have offered help a number of times, there is a tendency to stop making contact, not knowing what to say. This leads to social isolation and loss of support when this is most needed. We therefore recommended that people 'just say yes' to offers of help. Once this process has started, it then grows naturally over time. The important point is to understand what happens and get the process of network support started.

The value of this is illustrated by the story of one of our senior staff whose elderly father developed a terminal illness. Because of our project, he recommended that his mother just said yes to any offers of help. This meant that when a neighbour popped their head round the door, his mother's response was to ask for a pint of milk, even though she did not need it. When the neighbour returned, she stopped by for a cup of tea and a chat. This is a natural antidote to social isolation, loss of support and provides an ongoing presence for network development as the patient becomes less well.

Below are some quotes from carers and professionals which give a more qualitative view of the kinds of benefits people felt.

> Friends visited more frequently to sit with my partner to release me; a neighbour ended up cooking two meals and a cake every week; a relative who started off mainly telephoning began visiting. Overall, informal help probably doubled, and it wasn't asked for – it just came by itself.
>
> (Carer)

A friend used to come in once a week, another fortnightly. A relative came in daily and would do anything for either of us. I developed a system – there were formal carers coming in twice a day. I wanted to be a carer, but not for the personal side.

(Carer)

I never felt isolated – just the reverse – I sometimes felt overwhelmed: I had to reduce some professional carer services in order to restore time together.

(Carer)

I did not feel isolated as one particular network member would come as needed.

(Carer)

Accepting meals cooked by a friend for the first time.

(Community companion)

Sense of isolation and helplessness was altered entirely as carer had a point of contact that was available just to listen when things were getting too much.

(Community companion)

The input helped to coordinate social support that was already present.

(Referrer)

Able to use the people already known to him that wanted to be of help.

(Referrer)

The community companion helped the carer identify friends and colleagues within network who were willing and able to offer practical and/or emotional support.

(Referrer)

We started to use a form of a network map to see if this helped people visualise their networks and see the kind of support available. Although this proved to be more complex to facilitate than community companions liked, at times it seemed to have a degree of therapeutic impact. As one noted, 'Without doubt, it was good to sit down and do a "fundamental approach" with the mapping. At the time I was very scatter-brained.'

Bereavement support

Whereas most community companion relationships have continued after bereavement, none have lasted more than a month. Whilst we have created the opportunity for a more ongoing relationship, so far, the carers have not wanted to continue this. We are unclear at the moment as to why this is the case and will look at future patterns of contact as the project develops further.

Unanticipated outcomes

A mother who looked after her son told us that she felt isolated from her friends. People offered help at the outset, but she had said no as she did not want to be a burden. In addition, she had not felt like talking about her son's illness. She saw on reflection that this combination meant that it was difficult for her friends to find ways of supporting her and, over time, this increased her isolation.

From the elements outlined above, a key emergent element was the notion of the 'enabling environment'. Relationships with local community and government organisations were nurtured by the project coordinator from early on. What has emerged externally as a result of all this is a greater confidence by the hospice in interacting with community groups, a local authority keen to engage more with short-term and intensive carer needs, and social care commissioners and implementing agencies increasingly recognising the potential for network development in carer support generally in our area. As one of the latter recently noted, 'The concept of participatory network mapping was new to me and we are starting to think about ways in which we might be able to embed this type of approach in other areas of work.'

Lessons learned

Community companion training proved to be something of a dilemma. Our premise was that people who were bereaved and had cared for a loved one already had knowledge and insight, they would already be familiar with the fundamentals of the lived experience of being a carer, something we as professionals would not know. On the other hand, we were offering training in what our perception of being a carer was, tailored to a traditionally risk-averse corporate approach to volunteering. Fundamentally, our belief in the value of the tacit knowledge and skills of people experienced in their own bereavement and caring has been affirmed. It is possible to think of this as rather than the carer needing training, it is the professionals who have the greater training need in order to understand the lived experience of death, dying and loss.

Hospices are not necessarily the ideal place to be a starting point for community development work. We made sure that the cultural journey to becoming a community development organisation was part of our original project. Whilst we have come a long way, effort is constantly needed to maintain progress at all levels of the organisation. We have found that a significant advantage of developing the project from the hospice has meant that professionals have learnt to trust community development working with a real sense of partnership. If professional services and community groups do not work in partnership, silo-type working with lack of trust and understanding can develop.

Managing innovation has needed leadership, experience, vision, analysis and creativity, alongside a generous measure of carefully nurtured networking and consensus. Sustaining long-term, low-intensity activities may well be manageable with less human resources.

At the outset of the project, we had thought that the most significant part of our project was managing network development using community companions with quite complex methods. However, as we have mentioned, network development seems to be an organic process with its own momentum. The main issue is to implant the ideals and practice of simple network development throughout clinical staff and volunteer teams and then to allow it to grow on its own. The key part of the role of community companion is establishing relationships and providing emotional support and sewing simple seeds like the message to 'just say yes'. Network development is then more likely to be self-organising.

Although it is possible to conceptualise network development as being a separate function, in reality, companions fulfil a number of roles at the same time. Whilst we were starting the community companion networks project, the hospice started a related service of companion sitters. This service was primarily to spend time with patients, whether this was to provide a break for carers, provide companionship or to provide support for someone who had very limited social networks. Whilst the training for both projects was somewhat similar, the companion sitters had a more supervisory type training. It became apparent that the companion sitters performed many of the functions of the community companions. They naturally established relationships with the carers and asked after their welfare. It is then a small step to begin the process of network development when carers are feeling exhausted and overburdened.

It was further apparent that the volunteer coordinator of the companion sitters, who had been a carer herself, spoke to the carer at the time of the original referral. This commonality of experience naturally led to her asking about the welfare of the carer, and whether they felt that support would be helpful. When the companion sitters then first visited, both they and the carer were aware of the need for carer support and possible network development.

We therefore concluded that whilst we had a clear conceptual model for what we wanted to achieve at the onset of our project, the reality was that the multiple functions of patient and carer support by volunteers are naturally occurring phenomena that are interlinked.

Hopes for the future

Our mid-term evaluation provided a good opportunity to pause and reflect on our progress and our learning. We have reaffirmed our basic belief that people who have been through bereavement have a lot to offer carers and that it is perhaps the professionals who need education as much if not more than the companions.

Our experience has been that the reality of providing support is not neatly confined to separate roles. Rather, we are moving towards having companions who provide a variety of different kinds of support, including that of emotional support for the carer and enabling network development. Our aim is to offer all of our families the opportunity of having a companion from the point of referral onwards. Some of our companions believe that they are able to offer emotional support over and above that of professionals, in that being a professional can, for some people, be a barrier to openness. We are looking to develop our service so that the assessment and coordination of referrals, with matching to a more generic type of companion, will be done by volunteers. Training will become more based around supervision rather than a more didactic theoretical approach. Risk-aversion is problematic for any professional organisation and how the hospice is comfortably able to manage this remains an area for further exploration.

We have also drawn some inspiration from the recent national success of the 'Dementia friends' initiative. We hope that it might prove to be an appropriate analogy for a similar national movement of 'Carer friends' – of people who know how to sensitively and practically or emotionally support those around them with a heavy (even if welcome) caring role.

We are now much clearer about the functions or roles of emotional support for carers and how enhancing naturally occurring supportive networks can both have a tremendous positive impact on the experiences of death, dying and loss. They are experiences that communities have supported as a normal part of our evolution and existence. Professionalisation of care has led to something of a loss of these normal kinds of community support and we see our project as part of a larger movement in re-establishing it. To this end, we are now starting to work with businesses, schools and other organisations, as well as community groups, to develop and enhance naturally supportive caring networks at end of life. Communities occur wherever there are people, which is everywhere, whether this is inside formal organisations or informal gatherings in whichever circumstances. All of these provide an opportunity for community development.

The international compassionate communities movement, and Allan Kellehear specifically, are championing a movement to make every significant local government adopt a compassionate charter. We see our project as a bridge to developing such an initiative in our own catchment area, and hopefully providing a case study and inspiration for other community advocates to take up the challenge with their own areas.

Lastly, we have had many invitations and opportunities to share our learning along the way, and hope to inspire a new boost within the palliative care world, to take on the support of informal caring networks everywhere, in full, not token, partnership with ongoing (and necessary) clinical work.

References

Abel, J., Bowra, J., Walter, T. and Howarth, G. (2011) Compassionate community networks: supporting home dying. *BMJ Supportive and Palliative Care, 1*(2), 129–133.

Abel, J., Walter, T., Carey, L.B., Rosenberg, J., Noonan, K., Horsfall, D., et al. (2013) Circles of care: should community development redefine the practice of palliative care? *BMJ Supportive and Palliative Care, 3*(4), 383–388.

Burns, C.M., Abernethy, A.P., Dal Grande, E. and Currow, D.C. (2013) Uncovering an invisible network of direct caregivers at the end of life: a population study. *Palliative Medicine, 27*(7), 608–615.

Department of Health (DH). (2006) *Our Health, Our Care, Our Say : A New Direction for Community Services : Executive Summary*. White Paper. London: The Stationery Office.

Department of Health (DH). (2008) *End of Life Care Strategy: Promoting High Quality Care for All Adults at the End of Life*. London: DH.

Horsfall, D., Noonan, K., Leonard, R., NSW Cancer Council, University of Western Sydney and LifeCircle. (2012) Bringing Our Dying Home : Creating Community at End of Life, 2nd edn. Penrith, NSW: University of Western Sydney.

Kellehear, A. (2005) *Compassionate Cities*. London: Routledge.

Leonard, R., Horsfall, D. and Noonan, K. (2013) Identifying changes in the support networks of end-of-life carers using social network analysis. *BMJ Supportive and Palliative Care*. doi: 10.1136/bmjspcare-2012-000257

Network (National End of Life Care Intelligence Network – NEoLCIN) (2014a) End of Life Care CCG profiles. www.endoflifecare-intelligence.org.uk/profiles/CCGs/Place_of_Death/atlas.html (Accessed 11 February 2015).

Network (National End of Life Care Intelligence Network – NEoLCIN) (2014b) Proportion of deaths in usual place of residence. www.endoflifecare-intelligence.org.uk/data_sources/place_of_death (Accessed 11 February 2015).

3   Compassionate Communities in Shropshire, West Midlands, England

Paul Cronin

> No man is an island, entire of itself; every man is a piece of the continent, a part of the main. If a clod be washed away by the sea, Europe is the less, as well as if a promontory were, as well as if a manor of thy friend's or of thine own were: any man's death diminishes me, because I am involved in mankind, and therefore never send to know for whom the bells tolls; it tolls for thee.
>
> (John Donne, *Meditation XVII*)

In January 2010, Severn Hospice embarked upon a grand experiment – to work with local communities to develop their own free-standing volunteer networks to support the most frail and vulnerable in their midst – their own Compassionate Communities. The personal and professional significance of this development lies in my strong conviction that charitable hospices in the UK owe their very existence to the fact that, at some point in the past, a group of ordinary people felt so strongly about the standards of care at the end of people's lives that they came together to do something about it.

Compassionate Communities is but another example of that same response – citizens coming together to address a shortfall in the care of the most vulnerable amongst us. This time, however, the shortfall is one of social connectedness and its consequent implications for wellbeing and ill health. Just as Donne observed almost four hundred years ago, Compassionate Communities in Shropshire acknowledges that we are all defined and indeed sustained by the 'others' in our lives, who for so many of our older, frailer, sicker and dying neighbours are no longer there.

For me, Compassionate Communities is a reinterpretation and extension of hospice care for the twenty-first century and perfectly complements our 'day job' of providing superlative, specialist palliative care services. Furthermore, I believe to forget our roots is to distance ourselves from an extraordinary power and potential – the immense compassion, commitment and capacities of our fellow citizens.

Introduction

In the Shropshire model, a Compassionate Community is one in which citizens support frail and vulnerable people to remain active members of the community, with the aim of reducing social isolation and, in doing so, averting 'crisis' to which such isolation often reportedly leads.

It is a locally derived model developed in response to feedback from frail and vulnerable people. However, the importance of social connectedness in determining the level of subjectively experienced loneliness and consequent ill health is well documented.

In their introduction to *Loneliness: Human Nature and the Need for Social Connection*, Cacioppo and Patrick (2008: 5) state that:

> at any given time, roughly twenty per cent of individuals ... feel sufficiently isolated for it to be a major source of unhappiness in their lives. This finding becomes even more compelling when we consider that social isolation has an impact on health comparable to the effect of high blood pressure, lack of exercise, obesity or smoking.

The authors explore the factors impacting upon the subjective experience of loneliness which they evidence as significant causal factors in poor health and wellbeing.

Griffin (2010) in *The Lonely Society?* published by the Mental Health Foundation provides an overview of the impact of loneliness and concludes that:

> chronic loneliness can lead to serious physical and mental health problems. We have found that although loneliness is commonly experienced, it often carries a stigma and could become problematic if people are embarrassed to admit to it or seek help.

The report goes on to say: 'the problem of loneliness in society is a prompt to revitalise our communities and better integrate their members'. In a far-reaching list of recommendations, the commissioning of local services to establish peer support for people at risk of social isolation and the facilitation of face-to-face contact with at-risk people to bring them into wider groups and environments is proposed.

There is, therefore, compelling evidence that an individual's long-term health and wellbeing is significantly influenced by their subjective experience of loneliness which is, in part, determined by levels of social connectedness.

In addition, social connectedness is being increasingly indicated as a key factor in addressing future care and support needs arising from demographic change, and specifically within ageing populations in post-industrial society in Western Europe.

In his seminal work, *Compassionate Cities: Public Health and End-of-Life Care*, Allan Kellehear (2005) sets out the societal challenge presented by the increasing care needs of people at the end of life. He concludes that the prevailing view that a clinical service response is adequate in addressing future needs requires major re-examination. A future public health policy and practice response is important for complementing existing clinical services and this must include partnerships with communities: 'An adequate public health approach to end-of-life care must make central to its strategies, concepts that are health promoting, community building and partnership oriented' (p. 35).

Kellehear goes on to define the characteristics of a *compassionate city* as a vehicle in the delivery of such a public health approach. Central to the success of this approach is the notion of citizenship which 'recognises that people in modern society have a set of civil, political and social reciprocities with the key institutions in their society' (p. 47) 'a compassionate society is one where clinicians and community workers work together for the mutual benefit of each other and the community they serve' and at all times 'enhance the inherent abilities of a community to perform that care within the political and social constraints of its resources and vision' (p. 96).

These reciprocities appear to have been at least partially acknowledged by the UK government where the concept of the 'Big Society' was an early policy declaration by the Conservative–Liberal Democrat coalition government in 2010. This has as its aim the repositioning of the citizen and specifically the citizen volunteer in future services provision.

The UK government has also publically acknowledged the impact of social disconnectedness on health. David Halpern (2012), head of the Governmental Behavioural Insights Team, the so-called 'Nudge Unit' said:

> If you have got someone who loves you, someone you can talk to if you have got a problem, that is a more powerful predictor of whether you will be alive in 10 years, more than any other factor, certainly more than smoking.

Background to local development

Severn Hospice is the provider of specialist palliative care services to adults in Shropshire, Telford and Wrekin, and North Powys. As such it straddles the border between the West Midlands of England and mid-Wales. The population served by the hospice numbers some 500,000 people and the catchment area is typified by small to medium-sized towns set in large expanses of sparsely populated countryside.

Like other independent hospices throughout the UK, Severn Hospice has historically relied upon the contribution of large numbers of volunteers for the delivery of its core services. To illustrate this point, at the time of writing (October 2014), Severn Hospice co-ordinates and enjoys the support of 1,000 volunteers but employs just 350 paid staff.

In 2007, in preparation for an anticipated flu pandemic and as a buffer against projected staff sickness absence, Severn Hospice recruited, trained and deployed volunteers in roles historically fulfilled by paid staff. This positive experience in training and deploying volunteers in new roles provided the hospice with the confidence to consider the strategic development of new services utilising the significant skills and life experiences of volunteers. This had as its focus the support of hospice patients in their own communities, i.e. augmenting support for hospice patients still living in their domicile. Discussions with both hospice patients and people living with long-term conditions attending day centres in Shropshire during 2008–2009 revealed lack of opportunities for social contact and its negative impact on quality of life as a consistent theme. Furthermore lack of social support was frequently cited by patients and their families as a factor in the development of crises. As an outcome of these discussions, the development of community-based volunteers to befriend and promote social connectedness for patients and their carers was therefore indicated in future Severn Hospice strategy.

In 2009, as a consequence of this long history in voluntary services and its innovative strategy for the development of community-based volunteer services, Severn Hospice was selected by the then West Midlands Strategic Health Authority as a pilot site for the development of Compassionate Communities. Their brief to the pilot sites was simple and non-directive – to interpret the concepts set out in Kellehear's *Compassionate Cities* (2005) to raise awareness of the end of life issues in the local population and to develop model interventions to address local need which might be used for wider dissemination in other health and social care communities.

In the late summer of 2009 a discussion between Severn Hospice and general practitioners (GPs) from the Church Stretton Medical Practice revealed a potential opportunity to harness the capacity and skills of local volunteers in support of patients on the practice's register of those judged to be frail and vulnerable. In two open community meetings, members of the public were asked what their own priorities were for the town. They highlighted the needs of an ageing population (Church Stretton's demography is about ten years ahead of other parts of Shropshire) and the growing numbers of people experiencing social isolation and loneliness. The meetings concluded with broad support for the establishment of a local network of volunteers whose purpose would be to befriend clients identified from the frail and vulnerable register and to assist the client in augmenting their 'connectedness' with others in their community.

Therefore in the Shropshire model, a Compassionate Community (also known as Co-Co) is one in which citizens support frail and vulnerable people to remain active members of the community, with the aim of reducing social isolation and, in doing so, averting any 'crisis' to which such isolation often reportedly leads.

As such it is *not* a service provided by an organisation but rather a community development *supported* by Severn Hospice working in partnership with local medical practices. Severn Hospice supports the local community to develop and co-ordinate a network of volunteers whilst the medical practice acts to identify those with the greatest priority need in their practice population, secures informed consent from the client for volunteer support and acts as a point of reference for any concerns that the volunteer may have concerning the cared-for person's health and wellbeing.

The Co-Co network was launched in January 2010 in partnership with the Mayfair Centre, a local health and wellbeing centre in Church Stretton, when 20 volunteers received training in preparation for matching with a client. Since then over 80 Co-Co volunteers have been trained and deployed in the township.

As the aim of Co-Co in Shropshire is to support the expansion of compassionate activities within the whole community, the initial training provided is not only available to Co-Co volunteers but anyone in the community who feels they may benefit, e.g. life partners, informal carers, parish visitors linked to churches, etc.

Consistently, since the launch of Compassionate Communities in Church Stretton in 2010, the number of clients receiving regular support has ranged between 35 and 40 people.

Since the launch of the first Co-Co volunteer network, Severn Hospice, in partnership with local general medical practices, has supported 13 more communities to develop their own networks as illustrated in the map in Figure 3.1.

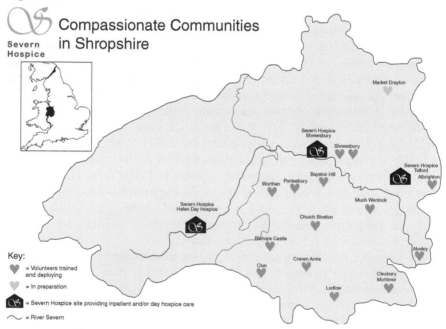

Figure 3.1 Compassionate Communities in Shropshire
Source: Copyright Paul Cronin.

It is worth exploring at this point what is meant by 'community' in the Shropshire model. In most instances, the community has been the local patients' group which exists to act as a forum for consultation with the local general medical practice. Therefore, in these instances, the 'community' is essentially the register of patients held by a particular general medical practice. Clearly this does not necessarily include all residents within a given community; however this approach does provide a recognisable division of local primary care services and a definitive 'footprint' upon which a network can be overlaid. Furthermore, in a rural county, the medical practice population often mirrors very closely the *resident* population of a village or small town.

However there are notable exceptions to this interpretation of community. For example, in the south west of the county, the Clun and Clun Valley Good Neighbours Group, which has provided *practical* support to local people for 20 years, e.g. running errands, dog walking, etc., asked Severn Hospice to assist them in developing a befriending service as an additional arm to their activities. This has enabled them to establish a 'Good Friends' service in addition to their 'Good Neighbours' support. In this instance, 'community' is defined by local residents working in partnership with *one or more* general practices.

How a Compassionate Community works

The structure of the Compassionate Communities model, being dependent upon the available time and capacities of volunteers, varies considerably from community to community. However the process through which volunteers are recruited, trained and deployed is similar and is aimed at assuring good practice and governance.

The process is set out in the flow diagram in Figure 3.2.

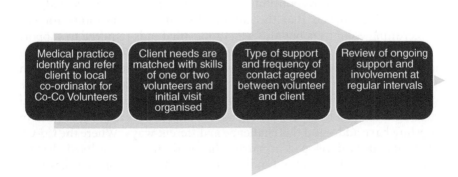

Figure 3.2 The process involved in the Compassionate Communities model

The GP identifies a patient (from here referred to as 'the client') who they feel may benefit from the social support of a volunteer. This is discussed with the client and informed consent for volunteer support is secured. The GP then makes the referral to a local co-ordinator who matches the client with a volunteer primarily on the basis of shared interests. The co-ordinator then arranges an initial meeting between the client and volunteer at which the frequency of visits is discussed and agreed. Volunteers are initially asked to visit once per week and to maintain telephone contact at other times during the remainder of the week. The frequency and nature of future contact is left for discussion between the client and volunteer with the sole aim of increasing the client's connectedness with their community.

In a charming example of innovation in partnership working, in one sparsely populated, rural community in the west of Shropshire, the co-ordinator, who is based in the local medical practice, matches the client with a volunteer in the way described above and then arranges for the local postal worker to introduce the volunteer to the client, thereby harnessing the deep trust felt for the rural postman and woman for even greater good!

Once visiting is underway a review is organised at an agreed frequency and typically every three months, to discuss whether the arrangement is meeting the client's needs.

In addition, clients and volunteers are encouraged to discuss any concerns they may have at any time with the local co-ordinator. This not only provides a check on the client–volunteer dynamic but has the added benefit of enabling the volunteer to alert the primary health care team via the co-ordinator to any significant changes in the health status of the client.

As an example, a volunteer visiting a client with enduring mental health issues, found her in a distressed state and confused over what medication she had taken or should have taken that morning. The co-ordinator, on being contacted by the client's volunteer, was able to arrange for the practice nurse to call in and arrange the medication in a daily pill organiser.

A key characteristic in the Shropshire approach to establishing a Co-Co network is to vest the responsibility for *resourcing* the network with the community. This means that the community takes responsibility for not only recruiting volunteers but also generating any funds required to support the network, e.g. volunteer travelling expenses, fees for hiring meeting places, etc. We believe this assumption of responsibility for resourcing is an important factor in ensuring the resilience and sustainability of the development, removing, as it does, the community's financial and psychological dependence upon external funding sources. Communities in Shropshire have addressed this challenge in different ways. Where the Co-Co network has been developed in partnership with an existing local charity, e.g. a good neighbours group, funding of the Co-Co development has been incorporated into the aims of the local charitable fundraising activity. In other examples, Co-Co supporters have organised regular coffee mornings which not only provide necessary funds but also provide a venue to which volunteers can take their clients and enhance their social connectedness. This has been particularly useful in sparsely populated, rural communities.

Audited outcomes

> We all decline physically sooner or later but loneliness can increase the angle of the downward slope. Conversely healthy connection can help slow the decline.
>
> (Cacioppo and Patrick, 2008: 12)

A year after the establishment of the first Compassionate Communities (Co-Co) volunteer network in Church Stretton, an audit of outcomes was undertaken by the then Shropshire Primary Care Trust. This simply compared the number of contacts the client initiated with local health services in the six months prior to volunteer support commencing, with the number in the six months following commencement.

A prediction that could be inferred from the above statement by Cacioppo and Patrick (2008) is that the enhanced connection provided by the volunteer might slow decline in health with a consequent reduction in the frequency of contacts with local health services.

The following graphs (Figures 3.3–3.8) summarise the number of contacts initiated by 38 clients with a range of local health services in the six months prior to deployment of a volunteer (left column) and the six months following deployment (right column).

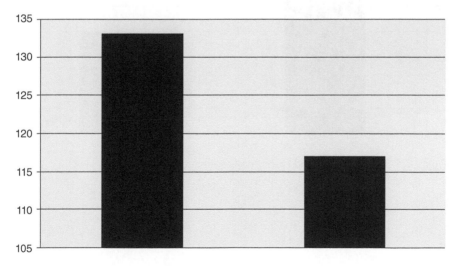

Figure 3.3 Total visits to practice

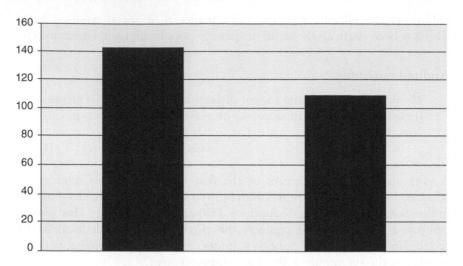

Figure 3.4 Total number of phone calls to the family doctor

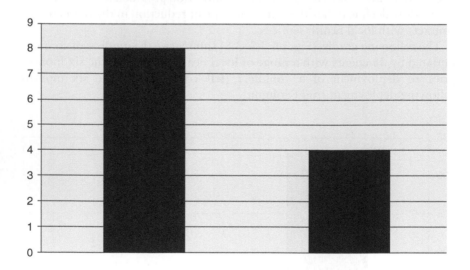

Figure 3.5 Total accident and emergency room attendances

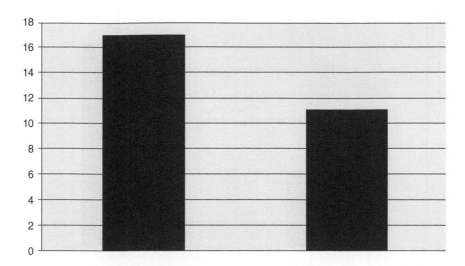

Figure 3.6 Total emergency hospital admissions

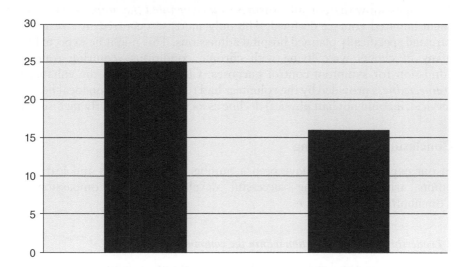

Figure 3.7 Total calls to/visits by out-of-hours deputising services

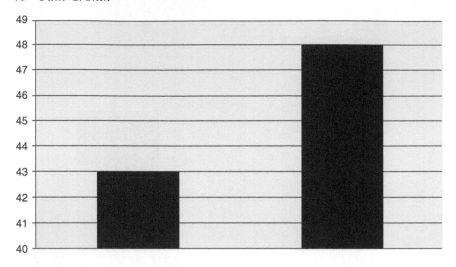

Figure 3.8 Total of planned hospital admissions

The graphs show that, on all measures of *unscheduled (i.e. unplanned)* care, client-initiated contact declined. The only increase occurred in *scheduled* care and specifically planned hospital admissions. This might be expected as many of clients were living with chronic conditions requiring routine admission for symptom control purposes. Clearly, whereas the enhanced *connectedness* provided by the volunteer had reduced the call on local health services, it could not halt physical decline associated with underlying disease.

Conclusions and learning

In our experience there have been a number of key factors and learning points arising from the successful development of Compassionate Communities in Shropshire.

1 Leadership and co-ordination within the community

The impetus for the development of a Co-Co volunteer network needs to be provided by a leader or leaders within the community itself. Such leadership has been provided in Shropshire by a variety of individuals but usually from those involved in other community initiatives such as community centres, patient groups or local good neighbour groups. This leadership not only provides the initial impetus for change but also a potential point for the co-ordination of volunteers once the network is set up. Currently in Shropshire the model of co-ordination ranges from paid workers employed by a local charity (Church Stretton), a paid or volunteer member of the General Practice reception staff (Worthen and Alveley, respectively) to co-ordination provided on a purely voluntary and independent basis (Clun and Clun Valley). In Bishops Castle, in a 'marriage' of community, general practice and local council resources and skills, referrals can be made to the local housing officer who is authorised to co-ordinate Co-Co volunteers as an extension to his housing duties.

The variety of 'solutions' to co-ordination is in itself a key learning point. Community development of this kind depends upon and is limited by the available capacity within the community in question – the constraints of 'resources and vision' alluded to by Kellehear (2005). Therefore the expectation needs to be that the 'solution' to co-ordination will, necessarily, be different in each setting because resources and vision are different. This very variety presents a challenge to clinical partners in the development where, for reasons of good governance and efficiency, uniformity in the delivery of clinical services is part of a shared 'institutional' experience.

2 Support for the community from a trusted and stable organisation

Griffin (2010) acknowledged the potential for commissioning of the voluntary sector for the provision of future services to tackle social isolation. It is our experience that a lead role for voluntary organisations in tackling social isolation and loneliness presents a number of unique advantages.

First, many local voluntary organisations themselves have been established through community action and, if they are also charities, already benefit from ongoing local support. Consequently, voluntary organisations tend to be trusted and relatively stable elements of a local community when compared to the perceived politicised and ever-changing governmental bodies, e.g. local councils, National Health Service, etc.

Second, the recruitment, development and deployment of volunteers are at the heart of the operational effectiveness and success of many voluntary organisations. Not only do volunteers provide capacity but their typical mature age and life experience present unique opportunities in establishing a community volunteer network.

3 Shared sovereignty in priority setting and planning

Like marriage, partnership with a community needs to be treated as a long-term commitment requiring compromise and the sharing of sovereignty over priorities and plans. This challenge should not be underestimated by professionals and their employing institutions, characterised as they are, by 'short-termism' in their policies and performance frameworks.

Furthermore it is our experience that ordinary citizens are very aware and impatient of such short-termism which, consequently, can present a serious obstacle to successful community engagement.

Kellehear (2005) highlights the challenge when he refers to individual's 'civil, political and social reciprocities with the key institutions'. In our view, local governmental organisations pursuing community development and community resilience as policy aims need to (i) accept the imperative of shared sovereignty with ordinary citizens in determining desired outcomes and (ii) develop performance frameworks to reflect the 'long-termism' and investment demanded by genuine community engagement.

4 Training, governance and indemnification

Arguably, other than under common law, there is no governance framework that applies to citizens volunteering outside of an organisational context. This presents a significant hurdle to overcome in supporting communities in setting up their own volunteer networks. However, in the absence of a formal organisational governance structure, virtual policy, procedural and governance arrangements need to be instilled to protect both the client and the volunteer. Under the Shropshire model this has a number of facets.

First, through provision of community-based training and education programmes, the *reasonable preparation* of citizens for a volunteering role. As the volunteers will be providing support to clients, many of whom will be frail, vulnerable and perhaps living with a long-term chronic illness, initial training focuses upon developing the volunteers' confidence in discussing challenging topics such as illness, death and dying; maintaining appropriate boundaries with the client; the need for strict confidentiality; and operating safety as a lone worker.

Second, in the Shropshire model, there is a minimum requirement for all volunteers to undergo formal enhanced disclosure under the current vetting and barring system. These are co-ordinated by and through Severn Hospice.

Third, we believe that regular review of the relationship undertaken separately with the client and volunteer by the local co-ordinator represents good governance practice.

Finally, we also believe that public liability insurance cover for volunteers is desirable.

There is no doubt, however, that even these minimum levels of assurance practice represent a significant obstacle to participation for some potential volunteers who, quite understandably, 'just want to support their neighbour', i.e. outside *any* governance framework.

5 Partnership with and close support of a general medical practice

In supporting the most frail and vulnerable in communities, close partnership working with the family doctor is an important facet of Compassionate Communities. This is not only for purposes of identifying those who would most benefit from support but also for securing their informed consent and acting as a point of reference for any concerns over the client's health. Acknowledging that volunteering itself can enrich a person's life, the GP may also play a key role in identifying those who might benefit from becoming a volunteer.

Furthermore, we also strongly believe that a Compassionate Community provides an opportunity to rewrite the 'covenant' between local citizens and local clinical services, providing, as it does, a vehicle for developing a long-term and qualitatively different relationship between the community and its general practice – the 'reciprocities' alluded to by Kellehear (2005).

6 Enlightened commissioning

Griffin (2010) recommends the commissioning of services that establish peer support for people at risk of social isolation, and good neighbour schemes that encourage neighbours to engage proactively with people at risk. Locally, Shropshire Clinical Commissioning Group (CCG) has gone further by placing development of Compassionate Communities as a central plank in their strategy for addressing the needs of people living with long-term conditions. This is enlightened commissioning. First, it places a public health approach central to its commissioning strategies. Second, through its partnership with Severn Hospice, the CCG has acknowledged the utility of the charitable/voluntary sector in leading strategic community development – a role governmental institutions would find difficult if not impossible to fulfil.

7 The future for Compassionate Communities in Shropshire

Compassionate Communities in Shropshire is demonstrating tangible benefits in increasing the social connectedness of the most frail and vulnerable within our communities. However we believe that we are still at the start of a journey. To enhance the impact of existing and future Co-Co networks the following actions are being targeted.

- *Increasing the number of Compassionate Communities in Shropshire and neighbouring districts* At the time of writing, there are 14 Compassionate Community developments in Shropshire. Our aim is to make volunteer support to enhance social connectedness available to anyone seeking it in every community in Shropshire. There is still some way to go in realising this aim.
- *Exploring opportunities for Compassionate Communities to provide a foundation upon which other compassionate activities are laid* The current model of Compassionate Communities in Shropshire provides the potential for (i) the involvement of more statutory and voluntary organisations in supporting the volunteers, e.g. gaining acceptance by Social Services and others of the volunteers' status in supporting and advocating for clients; and (ii) extending the range of compassionate activities undertaken by the volunteers within defined limits, e.g. provision of sitting services to enable carers to take breaks; bereavement support, etc.

- *Providing support for sustainability: co-ordinator learning sets* The first Compassionate Community in Shropshire was five years old in January 2015. Though there have been no instances of Co-Co networks failing, each faces similar challenges of recruiting and retaining adequate numbers of volunteers and the securing of sufficient resources to cover the inevitable running costs, e.g. travelling expenses for volunteers, etc. A variety of local solutions have been developed in the different communities, the knowledge of which might help the others. To this end a Co-Co co-ordinators learning set has been established which is hosted and facilitated by Severn Hospice on a quarterly basis. These have been highly evaluated by the co-ordinators in providing practical and moral support in addressing their common challenges.
- *Reaching the hard to reach: older men* Research has concluded that finding social activities that are acceptable to older men is a challenge. Older men are less likely to join groups and find making friends more difficult than older women (Age UK, 2014).

Just 10 per cent of clients supported by Compassionate Communities volunteers in Shropshire are men. The Age UK review (2014) concludes that:

> Befriending schemes have proved one of the more effective services for combating both isolation and loneliness, but they are best used in conjunction with other services. Group activities are particularly useful in helping older people out of loneliness and isolation.

We have reached the similar conclusion that a complementary method needs to be found to enhance social connectedness in older men and to this end we have initiated discussions with the emerging 'Men In Sheds in Shropshire' (MISIS) group aimed at co-ordinated action in communities where both Co-Co and MISIS are operating. MISIS has been inspired by the Men's Sheds movement originating in Australia, in which voluntary and social organisations provide hands-on activities for men aged 50 years of age and older. MISIS provides a space for men to meet, learn new skills and take part in activities with other men and is equipped with a range of workshop tools. MISIS aims to improve men's social connectedness, health and wellbeing as a by-product of these activities.

Conclusion

Compassionate Communities, as a movement in Shropshire, is now five years old. Though each year that passes sees more communities taking the step to create their own volunteer networks, there remains much to do.

Our aim must simply be to create a time when no one living in our community goes unsupported or 'unconnected'. As a student, my favourite graffito was 'No man is an island except Fred Madagascar'. Our experience of addressing the often invisible need of social disconnection and loneliness in Shropshire has shown us that even dear old Fred still needs friends.

References

Age UK (2014) *Evidence Review: Loneliness in Later Life*. London: Age UK.

Cacioppo, J.T. and Patrick, W. (2008) *Loneliness: Human Nature and the Need for Social Connection*. New York: Norton.

Donne, J. (1624) Devotions upon emergent occasions and several steps in my sickness. *Meditations XVII*. Folio Society edition, London 1997.

Griffin, J. (2010) *The Lonely Society?* London: Mental Health Foundation.

Halpern, D. (2012) Retire later to stop loneliness, says No. 10 adviser. BBC News website. www.bbc.co.uk/news/uk-politics-16980361

Kellehear, A. (2005) *Compassionate Cities: Public Health and End-of-Life Care*. London: Routledge.

4 Compassionate Communities in Sandwell, West Midlands, England

Manjula Patel

Murray Hall Community Trust is perhaps unusual as an end of life care provider, because the organisation works with children and adults across a diverse range of activities as well as supportive palliative care. The values of the charity involve addressing inequalities that impact people's health and wellbeing at any life stage including dying, death and loss. The charity is firmly embedded in a community development approach and it was through this channel that led the organisation to travel onto the path of supporting people at end of life. This chapter will highlight the background and context of the charity known locally as Murray Hall and the history of a community development approach in end of life care and to developing Compassionate Communities.

Community development approach to improving health and wellbeing

Sandwell Borough is part of the West Midland conurbation with a population of less than thirty thousand, the Indices of Multiple Deprivation (Department for Communities and Local Government, 2011) show the borough's average deprivation score ranked as 12th most deprived out of the total of 326 local authorities. In the early 1990s central government City Challenge funding was awarded to deprived areas, and in Sandwell, Tipton town received this investment creating literally hundreds of new projects. Historically, Tipton was in the heart of the industrial revolution and although there was rapid development the social and economic conditions were some of the worst in the country. The population of the town continued to have poor health outcomes and mortality rates were much higher than the national averages (Jacobs and Dutton, 2000).

It was during this City Challenge period that Murray Hall was formed and was established as a registered charity in 1994. Murray Hall's values are rooted in the principles of community development, and it aims to make a positive impact over the challenges of inequalities, to promote and support people in improving their health and wellbeing from early years to end of life through a community development approach. This is a broad aim because poverty affects all aspects of life, which has led the charity to being involved with many groups of people across different sectors on many diverse issues.

The concept of community development is not easily understood; the meaning of the term community is itself dependent on the context in which it is used. It is not uncommon for the term community to be used to relate to a locality and the classical term of community is coterminous and associated to a neighbourhood, village, small town or ethnicity (Mathie and Cunningham, 2003; Bhattacharyya, 2004). People have a sense of belonging to a community because of their own history to a place but there are other reasons as well. Elective belonging can be seen as nostalgic about social identity rather than just identity to one locality (Savage, 2008), but a sense of community can be associated to particular qualities expected within relationships, for example, by affiliation.

The essence of *community* could be portrayed as a sense of 'solidarity' a term originally used by Tonnies (1963) as a shared identity to a place, ideology or interest with a code of conduct or norms (Bhattacharyya, 2004). The term social capital is better known than solidarity; the characteristic of social capital includes a sense of local identity and solidarity, civil engagement and community networks, and the norm of trust and reciprocity (Campbell, 1999). Social capital is defined as consisting of 'trust' as social value, and trust can be described as the glue that holds communities together.

While the term community may encapsulate all of the above, *development* is described as 'agency', a modern term to foster choice aiming to achieve self-determination. Agency means that an individual has the capacity of a person to act as a self-conscious human being in the world: to take actions in the world around them.

From this understanding the purpose of community development is then conceptualised as the promotion of (community) solidarity and (development) agency that in part sets the agenda for community development (Bhattacharyya, 1995). Murray Hall's community development approach is to encourage and foster solutions to inequalities found in the erosion of solidarity and to nurture agency.

The Sandwell City Challenge health strategy recognised that the core issues of poverty need to be addressed to improve the health of the population. During the 1990s other initiatives included Sandwell gaining Health Action Zone status with the local health authority adopting a community health development approach for health improvements based on a model developed by Smithies and Webster (1998). The model comprises different elements and linking them together is key, as is working with community groups to increase participation.

Murray Hall was part of the mechanism to enable local people to contribute, and to suggest to policy makers how to tackle the local issues they faced and best meet local needs. The charity has a unique position of being connected at the grass roots, combined with being in a position to influence at strategic levels. The charity's work has been wide ranging and encompassed many creative projects and initiatives and has a history of developing innovative services that have gone on to become core services.

At the beginning of the millennium, and from being a key partner in many of the local developments, Murray Hall was in a position to contribute to the development of the National Health Service (NHS) Plan (Department of Health (DH), 2000). It was during this period that Murray Hall was one of the strategic partners in the development of a new health centre that brought together acute services, primary care, independent pharmacy, opticians and other community services. Murray Hall managed a health information point, a health café, community space and online learning all at the health centre, working closely with the local Public Health team to develop many different health initiatives.

Stepping into the world of palliative care

Towards the end of the twentieth century the health information point, which could be described as a physical library of health information, found people living with cancer were coming up to the information desk asking for help and support, not knowing where else to turn to. This alerted Murray Hall to consult with people living with cancer and identified with them gaps in many areas of support from diagnosis, treatment and towards the end of life. Unlike more affluent areas, Sandwell has never had a hospice, but has depended on other hospices from neighbouring boroughs for palliative care. Most hospices were established and are sustained with funding raised from public campaigns and most were set up to support people with terminal cancer prognosis.

Working with the community

Based on the identified needs, Murray Hall applied for funding from the New Opportunity Fund to set up a support project for people living with cancer and was successful in 2001 (it now supports people at end-stage of any illness). The name of the project, 'Bridges', was chosen by a carer who had cared for her dying husband and although their experience of clinical care was very good, they found there was a chasm between them and the health services. In hindsight it could not have been a better analogy, since it is very relevant as the service is a literal bridge for people to access support and care.

The involvement of service user and community members has been at the centre of developing the service to be person-centred, flexible and reliable. The service model includes making sure people have the information they need to make informed choices and decisions, are able to find emotional support when required, and practical support to enable them to remain at home, such as accessing equipment, care visits or shopping. All of these elements are interlinked and encompassed with spiritual support giving people the opportunity to consider the things that matter to them the most at this stage of their lives. Volunteers have been involved from the beginning, providing support in different ways, mostly visiting people with a life-limiting illness and/or their carers. Volunteer drivers play a crucial role in supporting people to access treatment and medical appointments.

Supporting people involves listening and we found people appreciated the opportunity to be able to tell us stories of their lives, about how the illness affects them, and about what matters to them the most. As narrators of their own stories people convey their values and discover for themselves their own meaning, most poignant at end of life. At about the same time as when Bridges started the NHS reform was being directed towards a patient-centred health care to be led by patients' needs, offering choice to move the balance of power, for patients to have a better experience of care (DH, 2000).

Intrinsic to our grass-roots approach, we developed a narrative-based assessment model to identify needs. Encouraging people to tell their story places them in the centre of the assessment and gives them control of what they want to express. Research has shown that narrative-based assessment is very accurate in identifying needs; but also in identifying unrecognised needs that people express as a worry or an anxiety not necessarily as a need because they do not perceive a solution. Enabling access to information and resource can be empowering, which is one of the principles of community development. Through the service we have supported, worked alongside and accompanied many people and their carers at end of life and these experiences have informed the development of the support we offer and continuously keep us anchored to the issues that people face on a daily basis.

In many ways because of Murray Hall's disposition to community development we were practising elements of a public health approach to palliative care before we began developing Compassionate Communities as a distinct project. Some of the initiatives we were involved with would now be considered to be under the banner of Compassionate Communities. This has included setting up a cancer self-help support group, which was initiated by service users expressing a desire to be in touch with others in similar circumstances to their own. We facilitated a consultation day where about 50 people attended and they set up the aims of the group to be aligned to their perceived needs. It was interesting that one of the requests for the group was not to just talk about cancer but to have 'fun' as well. That was over a decade ago and the group continues to meet. On average about 20 people attend each month, and we have volunteers who help to facilitate the group together with group members.

We have supported other groups to become established and increase their capacity to support people at end of life. One particular small charity was Tipton Listeners, offering people structured listening sessions to support people needing to talk through their problems with someone but not necessarily a counsellor. The support is offered by trained volunteers at local health centre facilities. However, we found many of the people we supported were unable to leave their home and so could not have access to a Listener. We therefore supported the charity with information and advice about home visiting, lone working and safeguards, to increase their capacity to support people at home, and over the years many people at end of life have benefited from this support.

Using the arts

We have found art in many different forms to be an important way of engaging, expressing and giving form to that which cannot be articulated in words alone. In 2003 in partnership with Sandwell Public Health we hosted an exhibition at the health centre called Bald Statements – Good Grief, a collection of alabaster sculptures depicting the facial expressions of loss and grief. It was the first time such art had been exhibited at the health centre for members of the public as well as professionals. The artist gave guided talks over the week about her own experiences of loss; many people associated with the emotions expressed in the sculptures.

At the beginning of the twenty-first century, dealing with death and dying as a natural stage of life very rarely made headline news, with the exception of stories of individuals who due to their own dying circumstances campaigned to change the law. During 2006 a national group, 'Well Being in Dying', was convened to explore ways of improving end of life experiences. The group acknowledged the value of narratives and recognised the limited number of stories of death and dying as a normal part of everyday life available to members of the public. Death and dying was still a hidden phenomenon, especially when the majority of people died in hospital settings. Together with another member of the group, the End of Life Care Lead for NHS Strategic Health Authority (SHA) West Midlands, and others we secured funding from the Arts Council for a story collecting project. We worked with a professional story teller, other artists, people who had a life-limiting illness, people who were dying and bereaved carers.

The stories that were collected gave an insight into the 'ordinary' experience of death, dying and living with loss and uncertainties. The story teller created a new story in the language of poetry and metaphors to capture the main themes of all the participants and their experiences. The compilation of stories accumulated in a book, *The First Primrose* (Whatton, 2008), which was made available on the website, in written form and as audible stories in MP3 files and CDs. The stories in different formats were distributed widely including to all the libraries in Sandwell as part of their resource for lending.

Reasons for developing Compassionate Communities

The *End of Life Care Strategy* (DH, 2008) includes a short section about society, acknowledging the need to engage with society to have open dialogue about death, dying and loss. The direction of travel for Murray Hall into end of life was from a value base of community development. As a non-clinical service we have achieved a high level of integration with clinical services and become a core community service for supporting people in the last year of life. The SHA End of Life Care Lead first brought to our attention the idea of Compassionate Cities and shortly after we heard Allan Kellehear (2005) present 'Compassionate Communities' at Teesside University. We instantly understood and identified with the concept; it was illuminating to hear about a non-clinical approach to end of life care, unlike the clinical perspective that had become the norm. The concept of Compassionate Communities gave us the opportunity to work closer with and re-empower the community in end of life care, reducing isolation and enabling more people to live out their lives at home.

The development of Compassionate Communities

In 2009 the SHA End of Life Care Lead, anticipating the need to source future care funded four organisations to explore the possibilities of a potential care workforce amongst the older population, and to pilot the development of Compassionate Communities. Murray Hall was one of the pilot sites and the other organisations were St Mary's Hospice in Birmingham, Kemp Hospice in Kidderminster and Severn Hospice in Shropshire. Each organisation's approach to developing Compassionate Communities was different and appropriate to their area. All four organisations met regularly together with the SHA End of Life Care Lead to learn from each other and share ideas.

Compassionate Communities conference

In Sandwell one of the first things we did was to liaise with the Public Health Director to support this new public health approach to end of life. Consequently, it was in partnership and with the support of Sandwell Primary Care Trust (PCT) Public Health that we organised a Compassionate Communities conference to promote the public health perspective to end of life care. The conference was titled 'Back to the Future' and the keynote speakers included: Allan Kellehear, University of Bath; John Middleton, Sandwell Public Health Director; and Malcolm Bailey, Murray Hall Community Trust CEO. The conference started with why the status quo of current provision was not an option for a number of reasons including demographic changes, the forecasted shortage of a workforce and individual choice.

   The aim of the conference was to: share knowledge about Compassionate Communities as the underlining principle for end of life care; enable an informed debate about the challenges of a Compassionate Communities approach; explore the concept and develop new ideas about better integration.

The conference included different artists, a story teller who had worked alongside people at end of life, a poetry reading that was commissioned especially for the event, and an end of life art-based organisation – Rosetta Life – previewed a film called *Night and Day* which features the life of a person (at end of life) in a day. In preparation for the conference we went out on the streets of the local town to ask people on film what they thought of compassion and community, and the short film was shown at the beginning of the conference as setting a context for the day. Most people filmed expressed a sense of belonging to a community.

The conference was held at a vibrant art centre – The Public – and over 100 people attended. We officially launched the campaign to recruit Compassionate Communities Champions, and one-third of the delegates signed up on the day, some as individuals and others as organisations. The conference achieved its aim and generated great enthusiasm to champion Compassionate Communities. A conference report was produced and is available on the website (wwwcompassionatecommunities.co.uk).

Compassionate Communities Development Worker

The original pilot funding provided the resource for a dedicated worker. A job description for a Compassionate Communities Development Worker was drawn up, which incorporated, maybe for the first time, community development skills equally with end of life care experience. Needless to say, we did not have any applicants at the beginning. We revised the job description and decided to major on the experience and skills required for community development, and this time we were successful in recruiting. The role was to engage with a wide range of groups in the community and to explore the scope of developing an elderly workforce; also, to network with community groups and organisations and liaise with others to create the momentum for developing Compassionate Communities.

The initial funding enabled us to make a great start with developing Compassionate Communities. The funding for the role of the first worker ended after two years. Soon after in 2012 we hosted another Compassionate Communities Development Worker for the Birmingham area, and in the same year we were awarded non-recurring funding from Sandwell PCT Public Health for another Compassionate Communities Worker for 18 months. It was not possible to secure the sustainability of these roles during the subsequent changes within the public sector with competing priorities. In 2012 in partnership with Dying Matters we carried out a mapping exercise of Compassionate Communities in England and we employed another person in this programme, so at one stage we had three Compassionate Communities Development Workers. All of them have embraced the concept and made great progress in pioneering and advancing our work in this area.

Methods

Naturally, we adopted a community development approach to developing Compassionate Communities and the various methods employed included: participatory, partnership working, end of life health promoting, and education.

Our approach to developing Compassionate Communities in Sandwell has evolved into a model that includes different elements as follows:

- Raising awareness of end of life issues within the community.
- Engaging with organisations, community groups and individuals to work towards increasing their capacity to offer practical support.
- Integrating the concept of Compassionate Communities at different levels.
- Supporting individuals and their carers to utilise support from their own social networks.

Compassionate Communities Champions

To keep the momentum going from the enthusiasm created at the conference we organised a series of workshops for Compassionate Communities Champions. The aim of the workshops was to create a shared understanding about the concept and together work towards developing Compassionate Communities. In the process we increased the Champions' confidence in talking about death and dying. The workshop outcomes were for them to use their own skills, experience and time to influence and promote the concept as a vital part of making the vision a reality, to get others to talk about it and to pass it on.

Together with the Champions we considered the language of death, dying and loss, and they were instrumental in the development of the dedicated website. They contributed from their own experiences and skills, they encouraged conversations to consider issues about end of life care with other people within their own social networks and contacts. They engaged with community groups and promoted the concept and engaged in conversation about end of life issues at health events. The Champions chose to participate in developing Compassionate Communities because they wholeheartedly supported it.

Raising awareness – health promotion

One of our first priority was to engage with as many community groups as possible, first to open up conversations about death, dying and loss, and then to share the concept of Compassionate Communities. The information-sharing sessions stimulated many conversations as people shared their own stories and concerns about death, dying and loss. The groups included:

coffee morning groups, daycare groups, older people's groups, community networks, dementia cafés, bereavement groups, self-help groups, church groups, children's centres, housing association groups, schools and volunteers. The conversations generated have been diverse with different groups and individuals; some have embraced the concept while others have found the subject of death and dying uncomfortable.

One of the challenges we identified with the Champions was the difficulty in communicating the concept of what a Compassionate Community would look like, so we sought to generate a virtual toolkit of different resources to help with explaining the concept, and as a way to engage with others. Stories have the ability to illustrate the concept of Compassionate Communities and the power to engage with people. Following a successful application a short film was commissioned and funded by the Media Trust to portray the experience of Compassionate Communities. We did not script the film but asked people who had experienced the support of Compassionate Communities to participate. The short edited film perfectly captures two stories that convey the compassion of people around them in the community. The film was shown on the community channel and is available to view online.

The film has been shown many times in different venues and every time it has generated a real connection to understanding the concept of Compassionate Communities. While the first film showed people on the receiving end of compassion, another short film was produced that captures the perspective of people in one community supporting an elderly neighbour. The film was a result of a Compassionate Communities Development Worker skilled in film making and photography engaging with communities (Ade Marsh Photography).

Another available resource was a photographic resource pack developed by the SHA End of Life Lead and the same photographer mentioned above. The pack includes many photographic images in different themes and is titled 'Saying the Unsayable'. It was designed to be used in group settings inviting people to reflect on the images and encourage dialogue about death, dying and loss.

The value of stories and narratives was evident as many people approached us to share their stories, and so it was a natural step to collect short stories of Compassionate Communities. A dedicated website was developed to communicate our aims to develop Compassionate Communities, to share the stories and to give access to other resources, information and news (www.compassionatecommunities.org.uk).

Engaging and partnerships

We engaged with many community groups and there were some who embraced the concept which led to partnership working to increase their capacity to support people with death, dying and loss. Below are examples of these partnerships that have developed ideas and increased the capacity of their organisations and within their community.

When supporting people in bereavement we know that some people need to rebuild their social network, which is not always easy. A bereavement support group is not for everyone, although the benefits of a 'safe place' to talk is important. The health gains from being able to walk and talk are evident and so we arranged to meet with the coordinator of the local ramblers group called Stride. They have a programme of weekly organised walks across the borough and we shared with them the idea of Compassionate Communities and how the walking groups may already include people living with loss but could involve others. The positive response led to further meetings, which led to us offering the walk leaders information-sharing sessions about grief, listening and responding to sadness. The training was to raise awareness and increase the understanding of grief as a natural response to living with loss. The Compassionate Communities logo was then used alongside all the other symbols for each walk programme indicating the inclusive approach. This means that information for bereavement support now includes joining the local rambling group.

Another charity that embraced the concept of Compassionate Communities was Salop Drive Market Garden, whose members were inspired to develop a project to create a healing garden. They recruited recently bereaved people to participate, and together they designed a garden at the market garden site to be a quiet place where people could sit and reflect. During springtime different community group members helped to dig and plant the garden. It is now a tranquil healing garden, an asset to the community. The original group continue to meet each week to maintain the garden and they welcome new people who would like to join them. A short film with the group members is available to view on the website.

Two of the Compassionate Communities Workers forged links with Ormiston Academy for an inter-generational project to work with a group of young people and adult members of their families on a photography project about death, dying and loss with the school. Tragically, a week after we started the project a pupil at the school died suddenly and the project became quiet poignant. The pupils involved others in their social network as they captured their images; the final photographs were accompanied with short narratives and were installed at a local art centre for public exhibition during Dying Matters week. Towards the end of the photography project we hosted a Warwick Art Centre play on tour about death and dying called *Passing On* at the academy with an after-show discussion.

The growing older population has been the focus of the Church of England Diocese of Lichfield with its action plan 'Age on Agenda', where Compassionate Communities has been part of the engagement. We were involved in the pilot of a national initiative called 'Grave Talk' similar to death cafés. Together with Staffordshire University we were involved in training the facilitators who were very enthusiastic and the feedback from the talks was very positive. The Diocese continues to work on Age on Agenda and currently we are contributing to their work towards 'Death Confident Congregations'.

Integration

A local end of life care strategy was developed as part of a Clinical Commissioning Group (CCG) Pathfinder pilot in 2011 working with a Locality Clinical Group – Healthworks, through a process of experience-led commissioning (www.experienceledcare.co.uk). The process generated a real commitment to person-centred care and to develop a co-produced strategy. One of the outcomes included Compassionate Communities being integral in the end of life care strategy; it was recognised that the concept needed to be embedded in end of life care. The strategy was approved in 2012 by the CCG.

Training

One of the actions from the local end of life care strategy was to embed narrative-based assessment and Compassionate Communities with health and social care professionals. In 2013 we were successful with obtaining funding from the NHS Workforce Deanery to provide training sessions for the health and social care professional workforce. Three training courses were delivered jointly between Murray Hall and St Giles Hospice Education to a cross-section of professionals supporting people at end of life from across health and social care organisations.

Supporting individuals

Narrative-based assessment involves listening to people: this involves asking individuals about their own informal care, their own social networks (assets) as part of their support structure. This gives them and the Bridges Care Coordinators together an understanding of what other support is required to enable them to remain within their own home towards the end of their lives. We are piloting an extension to these discussions with individuals to better understand their social networks and explore how we could encourage support to be fully utilised.

Sandwell Compassionate Communities today

From when we first started to develop Compassionate Communities we still have some of the original Compassionate Communities Champions actively involved with us to raise awareness within their social networks and we have recruited new Champions along the way. Some continue to support us in raising awareness about Compassionate Communities with community groups, while a few others are active carer/user members of the local end of life care group.

The majority of the communities groups in Sandwell have been made aware of death, dying and loss and the term Compassionate Communities, and we continue to raise awareness with community groups in a limited capacity. The dedicated website for Compassionate Communities continues to have information available to others, which includes the different short films, and is currently being reviewed.

Many of the organisations that we work with are all aware of our Compassionate Communities development work, which includes leaders within the local authority including Public Health, the Clinical Commissioning Group, housing associations and other third sector organisations. Many of the hospices we work with are keenly interested in Compassionate Communities and some are working with community groups in their own areas.

The healing garden is a valuable asset available to the community while the original group continues to meet and maintain it. The Stride rambling group continues to be available for people living with loss to access. The resources that have been developed, such as the photography exhibition collection, stories, network mapping display, posters and presentations continue to be used in different arenas.

The Bridges Support Service is in the early stages of working with individuals including carers to explore their own social support networks and how they can be utilised as needs arise. We are developing information literature to support this approach and we are eager to understand how it will support end of life care in the community.

It has been an achievement for the local stakeholders to recognise the concept of Compassionate Communities and incorporate it as a key element within the current local end of life care strategy. However, within a short time there have been many changes within the local health care organisations and we wait in anticipation of how the Compassionate Communities element of the strategy will be translated and implemented into practice.

The overview report of Compassionate Communities (Barry and Patel, 2013) highlights diverse approaches, and the balance required between a loose interpretation and an authentic approach with guiding principles to developing Compassionate Communities.

In 2009 we had the opportunity to share the concept of Compassionate Communities at a festival of ideas event with the Innovation Unit, where we had to pitch our idea to groups of people who were either investors, commissioners or business developers. It was similar to *Dragon's Den* where within a short time you pitch your ideas and then answer questions. Although there was lots of interest about the concept, it highlighted that without an evidence base it was not an attractive notion for funders to support.

The evaluation of the original Compassionate Communities pilot reported that the work was making an impact in raising awareness, which seems to be the case. The potential for a caring workforce amongst the elderly well was a possibility, and whether this becomes a reality remains to be seen. When we set out to develop Compassionate Communities we were aware that it would involve changing cultural norms, which would take time and has in some circumstances been challenging but mostly encouraging.

Raising awareness and providing the opportunities for dialogue about death, dying and loss enables people to share their own experiences, exchange thoughts and gain knowledge, which all contribute to reduce harm. A story that illustrates this is of one of the Compassionate Communities Champions whose increased confidence empowered her to have open discussions about a dying family member residing at a care home, and challenge the default position of being admitted to hospital. Instead she was instrumental in enabling the person to remain and die at their (care) home.

It has been very encouraging to have engaged conversations with community groups where the concept has found real traction and support. Some people have grasped the concept effortlessly as the role of the communities. In one group a woman shared for the first time a recent bereavement with the group, and by the end of the morning members of the group had offered support in different ways: it was Compassionate Communities in motion.

It has been very evident that the lack of research evidence into how a public health approach to palliative care can support people to die well at home has been a barrier to being taken seriously. Research in this area is growing and currently there are several studies being undertaken into the public health approach to palliative care. My own interest in this area has led to undertaking research with the University of Warwick: the study aims to explore how the different models of Compassionate Communities are understood and experienced; how cultural and social diversity is addressed within the concept; and how the practice and provision supports people dying at home.

The future

A research study by Horsefall et al. (2012) found that caring networks were strengthened and social capital increased as a result of being involved together caring for someone. It is not surprising when social capital consists of trust and reciprocity. However, the study concludes that social capital alone does not guarantee capacity building; community development requires the participation of individuals within the network to support people at end of life (Horsefall et al., 2012).

This takes me back to my initial point about the difficulty in understanding community development. Formal volunteering is part of community development and vitally important for voluntary sector organisations. Most voluntary organisations will have a volunteer governance framework to safeguard both service users and volunteers, so they are subject to checks, supervision and monitoring of activities. However, community development is more than formal volunteering, which is part of the service offer. It is different to capacity building in the community, which involves encouraging social networks to be utilised and generating more informal caring networks. If community capacity building becomes synonymous with just volunteering then we are in danger of disempowering the community.

Most recently, we have successfully secured joint funding from the local authority and Clinical Commissioning Group to pilot a project in two ward areas of Sandwell to support people over the age of 65 years. One of the aims of the project is to increase the community's capacity to support the elderly population, with such similar aims to the concept of Compassionate Communities we welcome this opportunity. It is encouraging if opportunities such as these are developing as there is real potential to join them up to end of life care as a natural step to Compassionate Communities.

References

Barry, V. and Patel, M. (2013) *An Overview of Compassionate Communities in England*. London: Murray Hall Community Trust; National Council for Palliative Care Dying Matters.

Bhattacharyya, J. (1995) Solidarity and agency: rethinking community development. *Human Organisation* 54(1): 60–69.

Bhattacharyya, J. (2004) Theorizing community development. *Journal of the Community Development Society* 34(2): 5–34.

Campbell, C. (1999) *Social Capital and Health*. London: Health Education Authority.

Department for Communities and Local Government (2011) *English Indices of Deprivation 2010*. London: DCLG.

Department of Health (DH) (2000) *NHS Plan*. London: HMSO.

Department of Health (DH) (2008) *End of Life Care Strategy*. London: DH.

Horsefall, D., Noonan, K. and Leonard, R. (2012) Bringing our dying home: how caring for someone at end of life builds social capital and develops compassionate communities. *Health Sociology Review* 21(4): 373–382.

Jacobs, B. and Dutton, C. (2000) Social and community issues. In: Roberts, P. and Skyes, H. (eds) *Urban Regeneration*. London: Sage.

Kellehear, A. (2005) *Compassionate Cities: Public Health and End-of-Life Care*. London: Routledge.

Mathie, A. and Cunningham, G. (2003) From clients to citizens: Asset-based Community Development as a strategy for community-driven development. *Development in Practice* 13(5): 474–486.

Savage, M. (2008) Histories, belonging, communities. *International Journal of Social Research Methodology* 11(2): 151–162.

Smithies, J. and Webster, G. (1998) *Community Involvement in Health*. Aldershot: Ashgate.

Tonnies, F. (1963) *Community and Society*, reprint edition, New York: Harper and Row.

Whatton, M. (2008) *The First Primrose*. West Midlands: Murray Hall Community Trust.

5 Community partnerships

A public health approach to ageing, death, dying and loss

Siobhan Horton, Rachel Zammit and Bie Nio Ong

> No one should suffer due to ignorance and lack of knowledge ... information is power; the knowledge to live a balanced life ... Providing relevant information is a matter of fairness and social justice.
>
> (participant from community consultation programme)

Specialist palliative care services in the UK, in particular those delivered in hospices and by Macmillan Cancer Support, hold a special place in the hearts and minds of many in the community. This elevated position has been forged by the profound effect and impact their care and support services have had at pivotal times in the lives of individuals and their social network.

The worldwide development of the hospice and palliative care movement in the late twentieth century has led to the growth of a body of 'professional' knowledge and skills (Stjernswärd and Gómez-Batiste, 2009). This is based on clinical expertise, but equally it is related to experiential knowledge and wisdom concerning the nature of the human condition, the inevitability of loss and death; and the human responses to those natural life events. Whilst palliative care organisations have made great strides in developing 'specialist' direct care services, until recently very little emphasis has been placed on their role in community development, such as empowering people and building community capacity around end of life issues and care (Kellehear, 1999, 2005).

This chapter describes the integration of a public health approach for end of life issues into the strategy of a hospice in Cheshire. We will argue that palliative care services have the imperative to release and strengthen the social potential of the communities they serve to address end of life issues. We will outline the conceptual and strategic development of a hospice-based public health initiative called the Cheshire Living Well, Dying Well Programme (CLWDW). In discussing the process from its inception to the current state we will detail the challenges encountered and lessons learned. The CLWDW Programme has been externally evaluated and the results will be referred to before conclusions are drawn and the future potential of an increasingly well-integrated public health programme within an end of life care strategy is considered.

The case for a public health approach to end of life issues in the UK

Taking a historical perspective the rise of scientific medicine has had a profound impact on how disease and natural, biological processes are perceived. The sociologist Jewson (1976) describes how the production of medical knowledge has moved from 'bed-side' medicine to 'laboratory' medicine. The consequence is that the 'sick-man' or patient is no longer viewed as an integrated whole-person but viewed as a 'network of bonds of microscopical particles' (Jewson, 1976: 225). In the medical cosmology of bedside medicine, where the patient's 'unique pattern of bodily events' including 'growth and decay' (p. 229), and the patient's contribution to decision making very being central, has been largely superseded by laboratory-based medicine where 'Living organisms and their ailments are conceptualised as law-like combinations of non-living elements and substances, life and death as physic-chemical processes' (p. 232). Consequently, the person is alienated from his/her own experience of illness and its implications. A similar shift has taken place with regard to death where the focus of modern medicine increasingly has moved to prolonging life and warding off death (Illich, 1975). With dying becoming the domain of medicine and science, a natural and planned for death is rendered the exception.

Despite the fact that death affects us all, contemporary attitudes to dying and loss reflect that society has lost touch with the natural life cycle; removed from everyday experience and consciousness (Conway, 2012). Many individuals in affluent countries do not want to confront the fact that there is no cure for mortality. Partly because the human lifespan has increased considerably in the last millennium death as the inevitable of outcome of life appears to pose an incongruity. One of the consequences of a 'death denying' attitude is that dying people are expected to fight to live rather than embrace the challenge of dying well (Rumbold, 2011). This may adversely affect their experience thus causing the dying and those close to them to feel isolated. Importantly, a UK General Public Survey in 2006 suggested that a minority of people (34 per cent) have spoken to friends or family about end of life wishes and preferences (ICM, 2006). Baseline research commissioned by Dying Matters Coalition in 2009 reveals that even fewer people (29 per cent) are talking about future wishes than in 2006 (Dying Matters, 2010). Yet, in apparent contradiction, the majority (68 per cent) reported being comfortable or fairly comfortable talking about death. Surprisingly, 70 per cent reported feeling confident about planning for end of life (Dying Matters, 2010). They view this issue as important and understand the need for such conversations, yet the majority of people are *not* having these conversations.

Do hospices disempower their community?

In the 1960s the hospice movement grew out of a desire that dying could be accepted as a normal life event and could be well supported with a whole system care approach (Clark et al., 2005). However, by the 1990s Kearney (1992) feared that the spiritual and social realms of the movement might be lost and care of the dying could be viewed as a segmented set of clinical services caring for the patient and those close to them separate from mainstream care. Kellehear (2005) argues that hospice and palliative care services became part of the alienation of the dying person from their community. He describes how they encouraged the shift of the idea about the responsibility of 'special' care of the dying from community-supported care to professional institutions. By marginalising the non-professional communities they were further disempowered. Community members began to believe the rhetoric of palliative care services thus losing sight of their compassionate contribution to the experience of the dying person and those close to them.

Early hospice leaders were skilled at influencing perceptions at an individual level, and in viewing death as personal. They lacked expertise in how to conceptualise social or political factors (Abel, 1986). Consequently research and policy work within the hospice sector rarely included community capacity building or empowering community development (Kellehear, 2005).

Key influences: policy, research and professional experience

An International Work Group on Death, Dying and Bereavement (2005) recommended a combined approach from public health and end of life care providers to forge an integrated community capacity-building approach to normalisation of dying, death and loss within society at large. The publication highlighted the need for permeability between direct service provision and public health and community development, and a need to engage with the public to promote open discussions about death and grief. It suggested that the goals of a public health palliative care approach were similar to health promotion in general, such as the provision of health education, information, policy making and change management. The innovative idea was that it would be possible to promote health in the face of death and grief.

In 2008, the UK Department of Health (DH) published its first national End of Life Care Strategy. It highlighted the relationship between death, dying and society. A chapter was included discussing the adverse consequences of a societal lack of openness about death and dying, causing unnecessary suffering through limiting communication about future wishes and preferences with loved ones (DH, 2008). The National Council for Palliative Care agreed to set up the Dying Matters Coalition to 'support changing knowledge, attitudes and behaviours towards dying, death and bereavement and through this to make "living and dying well" the norm'. (DH, 2008).

In 2010, NHS Northwest in its evaluation of a 'Dying Matters' series of events recommended that 'Palliative care service providers make links with Public Health to develop long term population wide thinking around healthy dying' (Khodabukus, 2010: 3).

Academic research shaped a 'new public health' paradigm articulating how a public health approach could shape a way of addressing death and loss. Kellehear's seminal works (1999, 2005) developed the theory and practice of health promotion within the context of the last phase of a person's life and within the lives of grief-stricken people around them. He argued that community care regarding matters of death, dying and loss preceded professional care, and that this approach views death and loss as everyone's responsibility. It should be considered as 'universal and normative' where community members have a significant and complementary role to professionals.

One of the authors (SH) argues from her professional perspective that suffering and its alleviation is a core concern for palliative care. Different cultures create difference personal and social responses to dying, death and bereavement, and she notes that in the UK many people are isolated in their end of life experience (DH, 2008; Dying Matters, 2010). This is contrasted with her experience of personal loss in rural Ireland, where death remains a community-based experience: the dying individual and those close to them are cared for and ministered to by the local community. Different community members contribute to the needs of the grieving families according to their skills, personal capabilities and availability.

When comparing how the two contrasting cultural contexts shaped people's experiences, the inevitability and universality of suffering in the face of death and loss was acknowledged. However it can be argued if meaningful and timely communication (verbal or non-verbal) was absent within the family setting and if the family was socially isolated from their community, the degree of suffering and separation experienced by all parties appeared to be intensified unnecessarily. According to Cassell (2009), 'Suffering is lonely' and withdraws the person from their social world. If the person's social world withdraws from them and their family and the family members withdraw from each other, unnecessary and avoidable suffering appear to be added to the experience of advancing illness, caregiving, death and bereavement.

In summary, the combination of policy shifts and academic research on the changing framework for public health and professional/personal experience were central influences in the development of the vision for CLWDW.

Initial community consultation

St Luke's (Cheshire) Hospice is located in the North West region of England. It is a medium size UK hospice. Since its inception 25 years ago it has held faithfulness to Cecily Saunders's vision for the modern hospice movement. Whilst excellent care with a commitment to education and research are commonly held as the hallmarks of Saunders's vision (Clark et al., 2005), St Luke's has also striven to be part of the social movement that Saunders articulated, that viewed death as a natural part of life and not a medical failure (Clemens et al., 2009). St Luke's endeavours to deliver an enabling model of hospice which strives through partnership working, education, service and community development to embody a hospice embedded in a public health and end of life care philosophy.

During 2009, St Luke's (Cheshire) Hospice articulated its strategic commitment to raising public awareness about dying, death and bereavement. This translated into the formulation of a community capacity-building approach in recognition of the limitations of the traditional health-care delivery models to the end of life experience. Individuals who represented community groups and voluntary sector organisations related to youth, older people, faith, social care, LGBT community, health and housing were approached in order to discuss a public health approach to end of life issues.

In spring 2010, the hospice employed an external facilitator from the Conversations for Life organisation (www.conversationsforlife.co.uk), to facilitate two workshops. Using an Asset-Based Community Development framework (Kretzmann and McKnight, 1993), attendees from the multi-sector organisations explored local issues and barriers. Community representatives were joined by members of the Strategic Health Authority, cancer networks, social and health care and a local Member of Parliament (MP) at the exploratory workshops.

Within the discussions two visions were articulated: first, the 'doable' vision focusing on the formulation and delivery of a public health programme that would support empowerment of the community through knowledge transfer from professional institutions to the local population. Through a community engagement programme individuals could be equipped with necessary life skills for a healthy engagement with ageing, dying and loss. The second vision, more a 'dream', was to initiate a local Compassionate Community programme (Kellehear, 2005) with the broader goal of using empowerment and education to strengthen communities and develop personal skills in caregiving of community members. Enhancing community capacity and resilience would lead to enhanced and appropriate support for individuals at the end of life, and in bereavement.

The conclusion of these consultation exercises identified an urgent need to engage with the local population to support its ability to conduct appropriate conversations within their social networks about end of life issues. This was considered necessary, not just when individuals were struck with serious illness but at any time in the life course. People suffered through lack of knowledge and were not empowered to act in ways that would serve them and their loved ones well in times of serious illness and death. Examples cited were making a will, or supporting a grieving neighbour.

The pragmatic outcome of the consultation was a commitment to develop an end of life public health approach. This would entail education about death and dying – including a healthy engagement with human mortality. Establishing this new approach needed dedicated skilled personnel who could lead, develop and facilitate delivery of the needed interventions.

Conversations were initiated with the Macmillan Cancer Support Development Manager about an application for a grant to employ a dedicated public health team to meet the needs identified through the community consultation. A successful application was made to Macmillan Cancer Support and two staff members were employed in May 2011: a Macmillan public health lead and a Macmillan public health worker. Close collaboration with the local public health teams was established from the outset, for example through their participation in the recruitment process.

The creation of the Cheshire Living Well Dying Well programme

The creation of CLWDW began with the appointment of a dedicated and experienced public health lead to centrally drive forward the agenda, ensuring that public health principles and practices were the core foundations of the work programme. This included the explicit assertion that the responsibility for health promotion is not confined to the health arena but includes all sectors, communities and individuals (Rosenberg and Yates, 2010; WHO, 1986, 1997; Institute of Medicine, 1988).

Tasked with making the strategic vision of an 'End of Life Public Health Approach' a reality, it was of paramount importance to one of the authors (RZ) that the vision and aims were articulated to ensure clarity of purpose and increase understanding in existing and future stakeholders. Ageing, dying and loss constitute cross-cutting issues and therefore a key part of this development process was to enable a multifaceted approach and embed this at strategic, operational and community levels. In addition, the recognition of the work programme providing structure and support for partners to collaborate towards achieving the shared aim was equally important.

Consultation with stakeholders resulted in agreement of the programme name (Cheshire Living Well, Dying Well) and buy-in to the vision and overarching aim of the work: *to improve health and wellbeing by supporting a change in knowledge, attitude and behaviour towards life, age, death and loss and through this make living well, ageing well, dying well and grieving well the norm.*

As the programme and partnership has continued to expand and develop the aim has subsequently been revised reflecting the learning of the Programme Lead, the team and crucially the Community Champions. This has supported clear and effective communications to enable, inspire and empower individuals, families and communities to recognise the benefits of making healthy choices regarding life, age, death and loss throughout the life course (Neuberger, 2013; SUPPORT Principal Investigators, 1995). The vision of the programme is driven by an underpinning belief that palliative care services have a role to play in the empowerment of the people and that a community development approach releases assets 'into' and 'out' of communities. A drive for knowledge transfer on many levels is key. Organisations such as St Luke's (Cheshire) Hospice and Macmillan Cancer Support are learning about the true nature and possibilities of working *with* not *on* communities.

Community partnerships: Cheshire Living Well, Dying Well

A participative CLWDW Partnership development process was undertaken to communicate the vision of the programme, to encourage cross-sectoral representation at all levels (strategic, operational and community) and to identify opportunities for individuals and organisations to add value to implementation. This process incorporated a range of activities including partnership development events, focus group work, virtual discussions, one-to-one meetings, briefings and presentations.

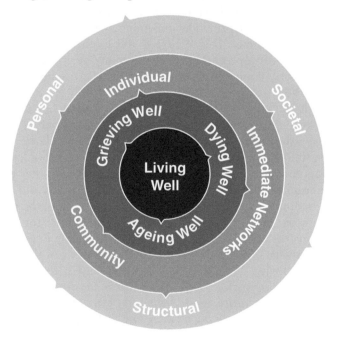

Figure 5.1 Visual concept model of the Cheshire Living Well, Dying Well public health programme

Source: Copyright Rachel Zammit, 2011.

Consideration of communication mechanisms and learning styles were integral to the programme and partnership development because commitment, skills and attributes of partnership/collaboration leadership are fundamental to achieving success (Oandasan and Reeves, 2005; Steenbergen and Ansari, 2003; Ansari et al., 2010). Moreover, the Programme Lead (RZ) utilised a visual concept model to convey the vision and concepts to the variety of potential community partners.

The central tenet of the model was 'living well', but that living well, ageing well, dying well and grieving well were all inextricably linked. In addition, it was to demonstrate that impact can occur from the outer layers of the circle inwards and equally from the reverse direction. For example, structural/policy changes related to bereavement will impact on individuals, families and communities and how they live, age, grieve and die. Equally, an individual who considers and records wishes for their remaining time and end of their life will have an impact on their own health and wellbeing and that of those close to them and how they live, age, grieve and die.

Following consultation the CLWDW Partnership structure was confirmed (reflecting partnership groups and representatives working at a strategic, operational, thematic and virtual level); branding was designed and adopted; partnership representatives were formally recognised as CLWDW Champions.

CLWDW Champions formally agreed the wording of the six strategic work areas and their objectives:

- *CLWDW Public Health Partnership and strategy development* (Embed a public health partnership approach to ageing, death, dying and loss at a local/regional/national level).
- *End of life (EOL) financial housekeeping and future planning* (Motivate and assist people to make plans, record wishes and have more open discussions about ageing, death, dying and loss).
- *Resource development* (Create and develop a toolkit of resources to enable effective and appropriate Cheshire Living Well, Dying Well public health interventions).
- *Public education, learning and development* (Raise awareness and increase knowledge and understanding as to why Living Well, Dying Well is a public health issue).
- *Compassionate Communities* (Build community capacity for end of life care via informal help from relatives and friends or via formalised volunteering).
- *Healthy workplace/business (Phase 2)* (Encourage workplaces/ businesses to review organisational approaches and recognise Living Well, Dying Well as a public health issue).

CLWDW Champions were identified and made pledges on a personal, professional and organisational level. The CLWDW Partnership was officially launched with an event in May 2012 that provided an opportunity to highlight the achievements of the programme and partnership activities. The broad-based structure encompasses the public, private, voluntary and community sectors and currently 176 CLWDW Champions represent 72 organisations.

The positive outcomes to date

The reach of the CLWDW programme has been commended as demonstrating work in a broad range of settings (Dinsdale et al., 2014). This innovative programme, unique in the UK, continues to demonstrate the wide-ranging health and wellbeing benefits through partnership working, and tackling this challenging agenda and unchartered public health territory. The programme has attracted contributions of funding and support from additional sources including the public health teams in Cheshire East and Cheshire West and Chester, and Skills for Care. The core programme team could therefore expand, resulting in the provision for additional support for Champions and enabling the volunteer team to grow.

Significant successes have been achieved to date: the programme has attracted national attention and the model has been presented at the House of Lords, consequently referred to as a model of good practice in Parliament and on a number of national and international platforms; the All-Party Parliamentary Group on Dying Well, 2011; Help the Hospices National Conference, 2012; International Public Health and Palliative Care Conference, 2013; Help the Hospices National Conference, 2013; Public Health England Annual Conference, 2014. One of the authors (RZ) was invited to present the programme at the recent 2014 Public Health England Annual Conference to share good practice and experience.

The formal evaluation undertaken by the Centre for Health and Social Evaluation at Teesside University has highlighted that the CLWDW community sessions have changed perceptions about ageing, dying and bereavement as individual and social experiences and not merely as medical or social-care led events (Dinsdale et al., 2014). CLWDW 'Raises the profile in local area of death and dying as a public health issue among a broad range of organisations not historically aligned to this agenda' (Dinsdale et al., 2014: 109).

In terms of influencing public health thinking CLWDW demonstrates a broadening of focus and that public health departments are open to considering their role across the life course: 'The team deserve credit for working towards a better understanding of what a public health approach to end of life might look like in practice and convincing others that this should be a legitimate part of the official public health agenda' (Dinsdale et al., 2014: 109).

A range of bespoke resources have been developed by the programme team and Champions (see website: www.cheshirelivingwelldyingwell.org.uk), including awareness and skills development sessions for community members. A research project was undertaken to establish effectiveness of one of the bespoke resources: community interventions to increase conversations and change behaviour about end of life issues (Abba, 2014). Some 64 events were held, with 676 attendees: 498 (74 per cent) were included at the baseline analysis, 478 (71 per cent) also completed a follow-up questionnaire immediately after the event, and 214 (32 per cent) gave permission for further follow-up.

At follow-up, 80 of the 133 participants who provided complete data (60 per cent) said they had either discussed their own end of life wishes or made some other change since the session and because of the session. This includes 58 (43 per cent) who talked about their own end of life wishes because of the session and 52 (39 per cent) who were able to undertake another action due to the event. These data support the use of community-based interventions to increase conversations about end of life wishes (Abba, 2014).

Across Cheshire, CLWDW has made significant progress in embedding public health principles into the local End of Life Care Framework. Local health commissioners and academic leads had the strategic vision and courage to support the initial concept and they championed the evolving message to be shared with key partners. In April 2014, CLWDW became part of a new organisation, the End of Life Partnership (EoLP) (www.eolp. org.uk), bringing it together with two existing programmes: one delivering education and professional development, the other supported service development. A research and evaluation programme was added to create a unique organisation that now offers a whole system approach with the aim to transform end of life experience and care to death and dying, from mainstream public health interventions to end of life care and bereavement. The EoLP's funding model has been secured from and is overseen by key local stakeholders from a wide range of organisations. The EoLP are currently waiting to hear the outcome of an expression of interest to become a Pathfinder Charter Community for Public Health England and the National Council for Palliative Care.

Challenges to be navigated

The programme has emerged through turbulent times. Changes in organisational boundaries and a major reorganisation in the NHS and local government have necessitated engagement in relationships with many new organisational champions (DH, 2010, 2011, 2012). This included clinical commissioning groups (CCGs), clinically led organisations responsible for commissioning local healthcare services (DH, 2011), and unitary authorities (UA), an administrative division of local government responsible for the provision of services including environmental and social care. Public health functions, resources and responsibilities moved from the NHS to UA in

2013 (DH, 2012). The authors have learned fast how to use levers and mechanisms within these new structures, and significant progress has been made in embedding the programme within one UA and associated CCGs, whilst progress with the other UA has been somewhat slower.

CLWDW has a small core team. The consequence of setting up an ambitious approach has led to the leaders feeling exhausted and overwhelmed at times, when trying to balance the need to pursue the organisational mission and maintain established relationships. Personal resilience is essential to survival as well as a supportive management and mentorship structure.

Healthcare professionals appeared more resistant to the programme and struggled with the concept of a public health approach to end of life issues. Initial conversations seemingly led to conceptual dissonance, where questions were raised like: Are you going to support staff to undertake Advance Care Plans with patients? What are you going to do to help (in care of patients)? CLWDW was interpreted as a direct line care service for patients and families. This was in contrast to members of the public, many of whom embraced its messages with apparent ease.

An unanticipated challenge came from colleagues in the hospice movement. Whilst hospice leaders appeared to be increasingly able to embrace the community volunteering aspect of a Compassionate Community model (Sallnow and Paul, 2014), interestingly some hospice leaders viewed the work of CLWDW as 'mission drift', that is losing sight of organisational mission and aligned responsibilities. Whilst others considered a hospice-embedded public health approach as a 'nice idea', but did not grasp that hospices could make a significant contribution to community development in a real and meaningful way. Conversely, Macmillan Cancer Support provided significant investment in the innovation, allowing specialist palliative care services to generate learning from integrating public health and palliative care experiential knowledge.

Finally, the programme has experienced significant challenges in establishing new Compassionate Community volunteer groups, for reasons such as the time-consuming nature of the process, and the need for flexible and specific skills required by team members to enable diverse engagement with community groups.

Insights learned to date

Leadership

Leading radical cultural change in relation to ageing, dying and bereavement is the underlying ambition of CLWDW. Key to achievement includes long-term strategic commitment; strong, dedicated and passionate leadership to translating a community aspiration and vision into a framework and strategy. Success is dependent on a public health approach becoming a strategic organisational priority with dedicated funded post/s. The leaders need to be strategists, and also opportunists who seize small or unexpected windows of opportunity to influence champions or stakeholders.

CLWDW evidences the leadership role for palliative care organisations such as hospices and Macmillan Cancer Support: hospices need to develop an understanding of their contribution to reducing unnecessary suffering at end of life caused by individual and social isolation and alienation from the life course. Hospices have failed to grasp the opportunity to influence through radical community engagement and development. CLWDW demonstrates the possibility to position ageing and end of life issues outside the healthcare arena for genuine change and embed this within the community.

Recruitment of staff members who are effective and inspiring communicators has proven to be of great importance. They will act as leaders in the field. It is imperative team members have a deeply embedded set of personal beliefs and values that death and loss are a natural and normal part of human life and it is possible to reduce morbidity related to this phase of life. If these beliefs and values are not deeply held, a team member is not able to deliver the message in a way that will overcome any of the more minor resistances in others as they will somehow use implicit disabling language that this topic area is too difficult and *maybe we should not really talk about it.*

What public health has to offer

The current era of public health often termed as 'The New Public Health' emerged in Britain during the 1970s and 1980s. This was a revised philosophy of public health that moved away from a medical model to a social model. With this new way of thinking, came the acknowledgement of the need to recognise environmental, social and personal factors in the promotion of health (Baggott, 2011). The Black Report commissioned in the 1970s was an indication of what would continue to be an increasing concern regarding health inequalities going forward. The importance of health as a 'fundamental human right and social goal' (Baggott, 2011: 54) was promoted, and the overall importance of strategy, legislation and policy as public health intervention measures was an integral part of the new public health ethos. The recognition that health is not an isolated issue and requires an inclusive response that cuts across sectors and disciplines was also a feature, which incorporated the challenge to professional dominance via encouragement of community engagement. This 'set the new public health apart from [all] previous [public health] initiatives' (Kellehear and Sallnow, 2012: 4).

CLWDW has grown in its understanding of the complex message required to normalise ageing, dying, death and loss, and the message needs to be 'life-course' centred. It has to 'normalise', be flexible and responsive, and people can access it 'upstream' when they are healthy and well. Engagement has to be targeted at the policy, organisational and individual level.

CLWDW has built upon public health expertise about segmentation and social marketing, in particular the knowledge that there are large numbers of people who may be receptive to a 'nudge' and who are willing and able to change attitudes and behaviours on the basis of appropriate information. The resources developed by the core programme team and the skills required to deliver them are intended to address this segment of the population. Furthermore, CLWDW supports Kellehear and Sallnow's (2012) argument that inter-sectoral cooperation between end of life care and mainstream public health services is imperative. Our approach highlights that political relationships and alliances can be forged across sectors; that a shared agenda and language can evolve; that a synthesis of an individual and population-based approach is possible; that moving institutional-based knowledge back into shared community-based knowledge is ethically correct. The drive to advance this new agenda is to reduce some preventable suffering and improve health and wellbeing related to end of life issues.

Creating a neutral and inclusive identity

The value and importance of creating a neutral and inclusive identity to support effective communication of the key messages became apparent to the Programme Lead (RZ) at an early stage. The consultation processes affirmed this with partnership representatives and Champions underlining the critical importance of clear branding, language and identity for the programme, team and Champions. Given that the CLWDW is dependent on a wide-ranging partnership approach, it has been important that the brand is not particularly aligned to either individual palliative care organisations or other particular local organisational bodies. St. Luke's (Cheshire) Hospice, Macmillan Cancer Support and the End of Life Partnership have adopted a flexible position to the traditional branding 'rules' of programme and team roles to enable public health and wellbeing and the CLWDW identity to remain in focus. In addition, it is recognised that continuous review is necessary to enable the programme team to engage with audiences in the most effective way.

The association of the programme to organisations with a strongly recognised emphasis to the provision of palliative care, cancer and end of life care services can have both positive and negative consequences on take up and understanding of the message. The key aims of the programme to support healthy engagement and action in relation to life, age, death and loss throughout the life course, often tends to be subsumed by assumptions about the predominant client groups to be supported. Champions and community members reported that a neutral identity was vital to ensure that individuals and communities did not automatically think this was 'not for them' and closing the door before considering initial discussion or exposure to the message. Moreover, one of the authors (RZ) notes that a need exists to use enabling and empowering communication mechanisms and language to 'sell' the approach initially as a 'door-opener' to overcome societal reticence in engaging with the core message (Gladwell, 2000; Thaler and Sunstein, 2009).

Future plans and conclusions

The programme has ambitions to promote a population-based approach to changing attitudes and behaviour in relation to latter parts of the life course. This programme aspires to be part of a movement for cultural and societal shifts in relation to future life planning that takes a pragmatic view on the normality and predictability of aging, death and loss. A challenge for the programme leaders is how to evaluate the outcome and impact of such a large-scale aim. The evaluation team poses this challenge by questioning how to evidence the slow steps of the programme's ambitions of a major cultural shift in ways of thinking and relating to end of life phase (Dinsdale et al., 2014).

The positioning of the Cheshire Living Well, Dying Well programme within the newly established organisation, the End of Life Partnership, will support the further growth of an interdisciplinary team with both public health expertise and palliative care expertise (demonstrating the interdependency of the two paradigms). The strong commitment to research and evaluation by the organisation and partners will also support continued exploration and development in the areas of evaluation, research and measurement of impact to enable increased understanding of what influences attitude and behaviour change within the field. Furthermore, this will support the continued development of the evidence base to demonstrate the wide-ranging health and wellbeing benefits that can be realised by working in partnership to tackle this challenging agenda and unchartered territory.

References

Abba, K. (2014) How can discussion of end-of-life preferences be encouraged and facilitated? Unpublished Doctoral Dissertation, University of Liverpool, Liverpool.

Abel, E.K. (1986) The hospice movement: institutionalising innovation. *International Journal of Health Services* 16(1): 71–85.

Ansari, W.E., Oskrochi, R. and Phillips, C.J. (2010) One size fits all partnerships? What explains community partnership leadership skills? *Health Promotion Practice* 11(4): 501–514.

Baggott, R. (2011) *Public Health: Policy and Politics*. 2nd ed. Basingstoke: Palgrave Macmillan.

Cassell, E.J. (2009) Suffering. In: Walsh, T.D., Caraceni, A.T., Fainsinger, R., Foley, K.M., Glare, P., Goh, C., et al. (eds) *Palliative Medicine*. Philadelphia, PA: Saunders Elsevier.

Clark, D., Small, N., Wright, M. Winslow, M. and Hughes, N. (2005) *A Little Bit of Heaven for the Few? An Oral History of the Modern Hospice Movement in United Kingdom*. Lancaster: Observatory Publications.

Clemens, K.E., Jasper, B. and Klaschik, E. (2009) The history of hospice. In: Walsh, D., Caraceni, A.T., Fainsinger, R., Foley, K.M., Glare, P., Goh, C., et al. (eds) *Palliative Medicine*. Philadelphia, PA: Saunders Elsevier.

Conway, S. (2012) Public health developments in palliative care services in the UK. In: Sallnow, L., Kumar, S. and Kellehear, A. (eds) *International Perspectives on Public Health and Palliative Care*. London: Routledge.

Department of Health (2008) *End of Life Strategy: Promoting High Quality Care for All Adults at End of Life*. London: HMSO.

Department of Health (2010) *Healthy Lives, Healthy People: Our Strategy for Public Health in England*. London: Department of Health.

Department of Health (2011) *Developing Clinical Commissioning Groups: Towards Authorisation*. London: Department of Health.

Department of Health (2012) *The New Role of Public Health in Local Authorities*. London: Department of Health.

Dinsdale, S., Carlebach, S., Hall, D. and Shucksmith, J. (2014) *An Evaluation of the Contribution of the Key Roles and Champions towards the Objectives of Cheshire Living Well, Dying Well Public Health Programme*. Centre for Health and Social Evaluation, Middlesbrough: Teesside University.

Dying Matters (2010) Research Baseline, Insights and Key Performance Indicators. June. www.dyingmatters.org

Gladwell, M. (2000) *The Tipping Point*. London: Abacus.

Illich, I. (1975) *Medical Nemesis, the Expropriation of Health*. London: Trinity Press/Calder & Boyars.

ICM (2006) How to have a good death: General Public Survey. March. Endemol for BBC. www.icmunlimited.com/media-centre/post/endemol-for-bbc-how-to-have-a-good-death-general-public-survey

Institute of Medicine (1988) *The Future of Public Health*. Washington, DC: National Academy Press.

International Work Group on Death, Dying and Bereavement (2005) Charter for normalisation of dying, death and loss. Draft statement. *Mortality* 10(2): 157–161.

Jewson, N.D. (1976) The disappearance of the sick-man from medical cosmology, 1770–1870. *Sociology* 10: 225–244.

Kearney, M. (1992) Palliative medicine – just another speciality? *Palliative Medicine* 6: 39–46.

Kellehear, A. (1999) *Health Promoting Palliative Care*. Oxford: Oxford University Press.

Kellehear, A. (2005) *Compassionate Cities: Public Health and End-of-Life Care*. London: Routledge.

Kellehear, A. and Sallnow, L. (2012) Public health and palliative care: an historical overview. In: Sallnow, L., Kumar, S. and Kellehear, A. (eds) *International Perspectives on Public Health and Palliative Care*. London: Routledge.

Khodabukus, A. (2010) *Dying Matters, Let's Talk about It*. Northwest Evaluation; Awareness Week, 15–21 March. NHS Northwest End of Life Operational Group.

Kretzmann, J.P. and McKnight, J.L (1993) *Building Communities from the Inside Out: A Path towards Finding and Mobilising a Community's Assets.* Evanston, IL: Asset–Based Community Development Institute.

Neuberger, J. (2013) *More Care, Less Pathway: A Review of the Liverpool Care Pathway.* London: Department of Health.

Oandasan, I. and Reeves, S. (2005) Key elements of interprofessional education. Part 2: Factors, processes and outcomes. *Journal of Interprofessional Care* 19(1): 39–48.

Rosenberg, J. and Yates, P.M. (2010) Health promotion in palliative care: the case for conceptual congruence. *Critical Public Health* 20(2): 201–210.

Rumbold, B. (2011) Health promoting palliative care and dying in old age. In: Gott, M. and Ingleton, C. (eds) *Living with Aging and Dying.* Oxford: Oxford University Press.

Sallnow, L. and Paul, S. (2014) Understanding community engagement in end-of-life care: developing conceptual clarity. *Critical Public Health* doi: 10.1080/09581596.2014.909582.

Steenbergen, G. and Ansari, W.E. (2003) *The Power of Partnership.* Geneva: WHO.

Stjernswärd, J. and Gómez-Batiste, X. (2009) Palliative medicine – the global perspective: closing the know-do gap. In: Walsh, D., Caraceni, A.T., Fainsinger, R., Foley, K.M., Glare, P., Goh, C., et al. (eds) *Palliative Medicine.* Philadelphia, PA: Saunders Elsevier.

SUPPORT Principal Investigators (1995) A controlled trial to improve care for seriously ill hospitalized patients: the Study to Understand Prognoses and Preferences for Outcomes and Risks of Treatments (SUPPORT). *JAMA* 274(20): 1591–1598. Reprinted in: Meier, D., Isaacs, S. and Hughes, R. (eds) (2010) *Palliative Care: Transforming the Care of Serious Illness.* pp. 185–204. San Francisco, CA: Jossey-Bass.

Thaler, R. and Sunstein, C. (2009) *Nudge: Improving Decisions about Health, Wealth and Happiness.* London: Penguin.

World Health Organisation (1986) *Ottawa Charter for Health Promotion, the Move towards a New Public Health.* Ottawa, Canada: WHO.

World Health Organisation (1997) *The Jakarta Declaration on Leading Health Promotion into the 21st Century.* Geneva: WHO.

Zammit, R.A. (2011) *Cheshire Living Well, Dying Well Public Health Programme: Visual Concept Model.* Cheshire: Cheshire LWDW Partnership.

6 The Compassionate City Charter

Inviting the cultural and social sectors into end of life care

Allan Kellehear

Over the last decade or so, the public health approach to end of life care has increasingly been adopted and advocated by international palliative care services. The earlier volume by Sallnow, Kumar and Kellehear (2012) showcasing practical examples of this approach demonstrates the breadth and diversity of this approach in several countries from around the world. My earlier work (Kellehear, 1999, 2005) has outlined the basic principles of this now well-known approach. These principles are: the basic recognition that there are limits to service provision; the recognition that health is more than tackling illness and disease and should also include the need to promote health and wellbeing at the end of life; the recognition that grief and loss are forever and need 'forever' styles of support and understanding; and, finally, that a public health approach to end of life care means to address the myriad and diverse social epidemiology of ageing, dying, death, loss and caregiving. Examples of this burden of morbidity and mortality include, but are not limited to, social isolation, despair, stigma and job loss to poor health, social rejection or withdrawal, and even suicide. In straightforward public health terms, all these social and health troubles are preventable or amenable to harm reduction and early intervention.

The social epidemiology of dying, death and loss highlights the gaps in our professional ability to cover all the bases of care. It reminds us that, no matter how 'good' palliative care can be, all health services are episodic and partial at best. Most of the time that we spend as ageing, dying, grieving or caregiving people is with our friends, family, work colleagues or simply interacting with other church-goers, shoppers or book club partners. Most of the time, we are at work, play or at home. Therefore, we need to place at least as much attention, effort and care innovation into these social spaces and experiences for our care at the end of life to have the best continuity and maximum quality. The best approach to health care and end of life care, therefore, must be a partnership between the efforts of formal health services and the concerted efforts of the rest of the community. This is no more or less than the recognition that end of life care is everyone's business.

To develop an action plan to go forward with these ideas has meant that we need to raise awareness about experiences at the end of life and of end of life care issues as social matters that we can all do something about and make a contribution toward. It also means working *with* rather than *on* communities, in other words, prioritizing community development as a process of mutual learning and needs identification between services and their communities. Finally, an action plan must include the creation of new policies to guide new behaviours in workplaces, schools, faith groups, high streets and social media, among other examples. In other words, a successful public health approach necessarily means inviting the cultural and social sectors of a community to actively participate in their own end of life care. Therefore, the aims of this chapter are to: argue for the need for a charter of social action in end of life care, to describe that charter in detail, to describe its social and political functions, and to suggest some basic ways by which we might implement this charter. Throughout the chapter it will be my contention that end of life care – like all health care – is a social and personal responsibility not simply a professional and health services responsibility. Community participation in end of life care is essential and it must come not solely from volunteer organizations and efforts but from the key social institutions of work, play and worship themselves. Only when this care becomes a civic responsibility will our efforts to adequately support each other become a reality.

The need for a charter

Most of the past efforts to create compassionate communities have been via the social processes of community engagement and community development. Key to the interest, involvement and success of many of these innovations has been the use of partnerships formed between palliative care services and community volunteers. In India, for example, Suresh Kumar's (2012) world-acclaimed community development programme – Neighbourhood Networks – has volunteers at the very heart of its support programmes whether these be university students, police officers, school teachers or farmers. Many of the programmes described in this current volume exhibit a similar approach, the shape of their programmes tempered by the idiosyncrasies of local history, culture and health services. We should applaud the extent to which these partnerships graduate into wholly independent coalitions of community support for ageing, dying, death, bereavement or caregiving, separate but affiliated with health and social services. However this style of services–to–community trajectory is only just beginning for many and is one that remains uncertain though hopeful. It is not clear, for example, how many of these experiments in engagement will remain dependent on health services effort and encouragement and how many will become self-driving community initiatives and developments.

Cultural and social sectors of a community that become involved via a community development approach initiated by their local palliative care service are very much based on how wide the local community development programme is capable of being as well as how large an area can be realistically covered and included in a palliative care community development programme. Even in the best case scenarios, such as the death education programmes led and facilitated by the Scottish Partnership for Palliative Care, which cultural and social sectors of different communities come under these influences is highly contingent. This depends highly on the reach of the social media and networks being driven by the different organizations participating in the roll-out and development of these death education programmes. Social and cultural coverage can be a 'hit and miss' affair. In the context of this pattern of opportunistic development and influence then, much public health effort to address the end of life care needs of communities wants for systematization – the need for a more systematic and comprehensive approach to 'community' remains a serious challenge. Furthermore, palliative care services often see the weight of responsibility and effort coming from themselves rather than the reverse, that is, looking to community to take leadership. Furthermore, in the context of the different sectors of community we often overlook or ignore 'the elephant' in the room of 'community' – local government.

Local governments are often (though not always) the key social institution in a community – City Hall, Town Hall, or Parish Council. Often the Mayor's office have major networks, partnerships or representation from employers, faith groups, museums or galleries, newspapers, radio or television, and social media, or from schools and local universities, aged care facilities, shopping and sports villages, and other leisure associations. Collectively these networks represent major groups of employees, students, parents, participants, shoppers, listeners or readers and any policy development in end of life care emanating from these networks will directly affect all these different constituencies. The same is true of churches and temples in a large town or city, or even the town's largest employer group. It is to these large political and social organizations that a Charter for Action is best adopted and employed for such organizations so that public health leadership does not become or remain the sole responsibility of the local health service. Furthermore, the promotion of a charter helps identify the key sectors of any community that need to be targeted for specific social action in end of life care.

Finally, just as there are Healthy Cities around the world endorsed and supported by the World Health Organization so too there can be Compassionate Cities supported by local or international palliative care organizations. The Compassionate City Charter is designed to promote leadership in end of life care that actively invites the cultural and social sectors of any society to take its place in this important human experience.

Introducing the charter

I introduce the charter at the centre of this chapter's discussion. This is a declaration of commitment, to be taken up by local government and or other peak community bodies, that commits that organization to a series of social changes within their community. Although some organizations (usually workplaces) have currently used the charter to bring changes to their micro-community, the charter was designed to be employed over a significant geo-political area such as a village, town or city. As such, the charter speaks to changes to the policy interest and development in schools, workplaces, trade unions, local government, churches/temples, as well as hospices/care homes. The expectation is that these former organizations will introduce collaborations between their internal constituents (students/teachers/parents or workers/managers/owners or patients/families/carers) to create formal organizational policies for dying, death and loss and grief. Obviously these will sit alongside existing policies about bullying, sexual harassment, sick leave or workplace safety and extend and complement these. As with many of these other policies, the new policies on dying, death and loss and grief will be 'living documents', that is to say, they will be subject to revisions and iterations based on lessons learnt from ongoing experiences of dying, death and grief and loss encountered within these organizations. Clearly, an annual review of these policies is highly recommended.

There are also several other events-related commitments that those who commit to the charter need to accommodate. These include an incentives scheme of awards and public recognition events that help foster and encourage individuals and organizations within a community to strive for greater compassionate responses toward others within their sphere of influence. A memorial parade – much like those we have all seen in gay and lesbian pride marches or in annual veterans day marches – is also encouraged to bring different parts of the community together to remember their dead. A short story or art competition encourages the creative arts community to support people not only in remembering their losses, celebrating their carers, but also assisting in reversing the disenfranchised position of those living with a life-limiting illness, long-term caregiving and bereavement.

The charter also reminds the committing organization of the importance of addressing end of life care needs and experiences through the lens of social, sexual, religious and cultural diversity, and asserts the needs of two frequently overlooked groups – the homeless and imprisoned. All end of life care policies of worth must be socially inclusive. Finally, as a reminder that communities are complex, diverse and constantly changing, it is incumbent upon all those who commit to the charter to critically reflect upon those they may have overlooked and to expand the work of compassionate care to those groups. Therefore the charter ends with a commitment to include one more social or cultural sector of the community to its policy development and drive each year. The Compassionate City Charter is reproduced in the box.

The Compassionate City

Charter

Compassionate Cities are communities that recognize that all natural cycles of sickness and health, birth and death, and love and loss occur everyday within the orbits of their institutions and regular activities. A compassionate city is a community that recognizes that care for one another at times of crisis and loss is not simply a task solely for health and social services but is everyone's responsibility.

Compassionate Cities are communities that publicly encourage, facilitate, support and celebrate care for one another during life's most testing moments and experiences, especially those pertaining to life-threatening and life-limiting illness, chronic disability, frail ageing and dementia, grief and bereavement, and the trials and burdens of long-term care. Though local government strives to maintain and strengthen quality services for the most fragile and vulnerable in our midst, those persons are not the limits of our experience of fragility and vulnerability. Serious personal crises of illness, dying, death and loss may visit any of us, at any time during the normal course of our lives. A compassionate city is a community that squarely recognizes and addresses this social fact.

Through auspices of the Mayor's office a compassionate city will – by public marketing and advertising, by use of the cities network and influences, by dint of collaboration and cooperation, in partnership with social media and its own offices – develop and support the following 13 social changes to the city's key institutions and activities.

- Our *schools* will have annually reviewed policies or guidance documents for dying, death, loss and care
- Our *workplaces* will have annually reviewed policies or guidance documents for dying, death, loss and care
- Our *trade unions* will have annually reviewed policies or guidance documents for dying, death, loss and care
- Our *churches and temples* will have at least one dedicated group for end of life care support
- Our city's *hospices* and *nursing homes* will have a community development programme involving local area citizens in end of life care activities and programmes
- Our city's major *museums and art galleries* will hold annual exhibitions on the experiences of ageing, dying, death, loss or care

- Our city will host *an annual peacetime memorial parade* representing the major sectors of human loss outside military campaigns – cancer, motor neuron disease, AIDS, child loss, suicide survivors, animal companion loss, widowhood, industrial and vehicle accidents, the loss of emergency workers and all end of life care personnel, etc.

- Our city will create *an incentives scheme* to celebrate and highlight the most creative compassionate organization, event and individual/s. The scheme will take the form of an annual award administered by a committee drawn from the end of life care sector. A 'Mayor's Prize' will recognize individual/s for that year who most exemplify the city's values of compassionate care

- Our city will publicly showcase, in print and in social media, our *local government policies*, services, funding opportunities, partnerships and public events that address 'our compassionate concerns' with living with ageing, life-threatening and life-limiting illness, loss and bereavement, and long-term caring. All end of life care-related services within the city limits will be encouraged to distribute this material or these web links including veterinarians and funeral organizations

- Our city will work with local social or print media to encourage an *annual city-wide short story or art competition* that helps raise awareness of ageing, dying, death, loss or caring

- All our compassionate policies and services, and the policies and practices of our official compassionate partners and alliances, will demonstrate an understanding of how *diversity* shapes the experience of ageing, dying, death, loss and care – through ethnic, religious, gendered and sexual identity and through the social experiences of poverty, inequality and disenfranchisement.

- We will seek to encourage and to invite evidence that institutions for the *homeless and the imprisoned* have support plans in place for end of life care and loss and bereavement.

- Our city will establish and review these targets and goals in the first two years and thereafter will *add one more sector annually* to our action plans for a compassionate city – e.g. hospitals, further and higher education, charities, community and voluntary organizations, police and emergency services, and so on.

> This charter represents a commitment by the city to embrace a view of health and wellbeing that embraces social empathy, reminding its inhabitants and all who would view us from beyond its borders that 'compassion' means to embrace mutual sharing. A city is not merely a place to work and access services but equally a place to enjoy support in the safety and protection of each other's company, even to the end of our days.
>
> © Allan Kellehear

Social and political functions of the charter

The Compassionate City Charter lies at the heart of the recently published 'toolkit' for Public Health England (PHE). *Public Health Approaches to End of Life Care: A Toolkit* (Karapliagou and Kellehear, 2014) is designed as a briefing document for those who are not familiar with the public health approach to end of life care. It includes information on the application of health promotion, health education, community engagement and community development to the social epidemiology of ageing, dying, death, loss and grief. The Compassionate City Charter is promoted in that national toolkit and together they are located on the current website of the National Council for Palliative Care (UK). The Compassionate City Charter has a number of important functions for the promotion of a public health approach to end of life care. These are:

1   *Educating/raising awareness `about possibilities and responsibilities*
    When most people think about a 'societal' or 'community' approach to end of life care they often think in terms of a collection of individuals or perhaps a business and shopping district and the outlying residential areas. Seldom do people think in terms of the sociological anatomy of a community. The charter highlights the key 'bones', so to speak, of most communities and lists these as important targets for influence and change – local government, churches/temples, schools, workplaces, cultural centres, and centres of communication and information. The charter also highlights new possibilities from old taken-for-granted social events and activities – short story competitions, award rituals or festivals and parades — as potential conduits for change, social cohesion and education. Finally, the charter reminds us about diversity and marginality within all communities and the need for social inclusion and justice in life and at the end of life.

2   *Promoting social innovations and collective responses*
    Within each of the sectors identified in the charter and within each call for action within each sector the question of how to proceed is raised.

Within schools or workplaces, for example, the call for policy development to shape our responses to dying, death and loss is a call for innovation and collective action. It is not a call for top-down managerial action by those who daily regulate these sites. Rather, the charter asks all those in those sites to come together to discuss their common experiences in the face of mortality and to develop guidelines that both reflect that experience and may provide principles for support, empathy and change within those sites that will aid future encounters with mortal illness, death or loss. Re-looking at the public events and rituals within each community and asking how these support our lives – even in the face of death – is to prompt innovation and change by making these events and rituals inclusive of all of life's most important experiences

3   *Mobilizing local political and social action*

The charter is also crucial to the shift away from a health and social services mentality to one steeped in civic understanding. Health care, social care and end of life care are not simply services provided by professionals. Care in all its meanings is also a community responsibility, and that is why we have laws governing the safety of employees, students, shoppers, commuters, prisoners or passengers to name only a brief set of everyday roles we all share. Our experiences of dying, death and loss have only recently been recognized as a set of civic responsibilities. In England over 500,000 people die every year. If it is reasonable to assume that most of these people have left three or four people bereaved and most of the illness-related deaths have had a period of care from family or friends then it is equally safe to assume that at least 2 million people *annually* are adversely affected by dying, death, loss and caregiving. No national health service can reasonably be expected to address this toll alone. Health services are not enough. Just as it is crucial for everyone – workplaces, schools or newspapers – to play some role in the promotion of health and wellbeing in a community so it is equally important to promote that health and wellbeing at the end of life. End of life care must be a target for political and social action if we are to transform it from episodic health service rescue to a seamless health service–community partnership.

4   *Creating new alliances for end of life care*

To create a transformation that would provide continuity of care for ageing, dying and bereavement we need a social system that relies on the health services to help us in crisis and in complexity but to have support outside of these times and circumstances. This means we need to forge new alliances around us. We need to make our daily work and play environments responsive to our most testing times and needs. To do this we need to look to each other, to our workplaces or schools – not simply for their taken-for-granted support in health and safety, or in environmental waste and conservation, but also in terms of our end of life care requirements. Just as we expect to learn about the meaning of embodiment, love, beauty or nature through art (e.g. 'Art for the Broken Heart') and literature (e.g. 'Scripts for an Ending') so too we should expect to learn about death, dying and loss through these mediums. Just as we can share a joke or a rumour via Twitter or Facebook we should also look to see how these communities and networks might work to support us in ageing, dying or loss. As long as many people continue to think of 'dying' as an illness-related experience unconnected or unrelated to the trauma of traffic accidents or suicide the complexity of the human experience of death and loss will escape most of us. Equally, the potential for broader social empathy and exchange is lost through this type of 'othering' of mortal experience. The practice wisdom of veterinarian experience with grieving owners of animal companions is rarely connected to the experience of those who work in the funeral industry, and neither sectors pool their experience with hospice or aged care workers, and yet these are support synergies we rarely put to good use.

5   *The charter as a fillip for national change*

Finally, the charter reminds us of two geo-political facts. First, governments the world over now see 'care of the dying' mainly in health service terms and *not* in social service or community terms. Second, that palliative care services continue to view their mission and their primary role in bedside care terms. While these two views continue to intersect and exaggerate each other's impact, end of life care as a civic responsibility remains eclipsed and in the political shadows. The charter represents the thin end of a wedge that may overturn this narrow line of modern but recent thinking. The charter serves to alert those who read it that end of life care cannot continue to be seen as a narrow speciality of health services alone. People who live with a life-limiting illness spend most of their time away from professional care and in their communities doing what they normally do. Bereaved people are everywhere and do not necessarily need services but that doesn't mean they do not need ongoing support. And loneliness and social isolation are on the increase (Kellehear, 2009) and has important consequences not only for the individuals themselves but also the communities in which they live. The epidemiological and demographic figures behind these simple statements demand a national response and the charter is a practical and grass-roots step to address this deficiency.

The future

Obviously, there are two major ways the charter can be implemented. First, the charter can be implemented as part of an ongoing community development programme already underway by a palliative care service. The other major way is for individuals within social care or cultural organizations to take the charter and advocate its use by their local government, church/temple organization or large business. At the time of writing, there are several initiatives that represent just these kinds of efforts. In the UK, several palliative care organizations – some hospices and some parts of Public Health England and/or the NHS – are advocating the charter to local governments in their geographical areas. As part of the implementation plans of Public Health England there has also been a call for six regions to 'field trial' the public health palliative care toolkit and it may also be the case that these field trials will result in the uptake of the charter by local governments in the regions hosting the trials.

Currently there is significant interest in the charter's uptake with ongoing discussion about methodology (how to do this) and accreditation (who and how will the charter be recognized as being 'implemented'). The newly established association Public Health Palliative Care International will consider advocating for adoption of the charter by local governments with the aim of encouraging them to take up its policy and action challenges. Health and Wellbeing Boards in England are also beginning to take an interest in what role they might play in the social and cultural dimensions of end of life care and the charter has potential to provide guidance for these organizations as well. But these are early days. The future for implementation possibilities, advocacy by hospices, residential care communities, community health centres or Health and Wellbeing Boards, uptake by Mayoral offices, will continue to be important drivers and facilitators for the implementation of the charter.

However, at the very least, the charter may also act as a guide for incremental local action – taking one piece at a time to showcase the social value of specific social actions on community support in this area, for example, by creating an annual compassionate festival/parade or 'Art for the Broken Heart' exhibition. It may be that not all communities wish to be bound by 'a charter' endorsed or 'accredited' by an external body and that has certainly been the experience of the WHO Healthy Cities movement. Although many cities do opt for recognition of 'healthy city' status from WHO many others do not, but this does not mean they do not aspire to create 'healthy' environments for their citizens. In just this same way, some communities may wish to strive for the basic principles of support and empathy at the end of life and use the charter as a guide to specific social actions that can attract great support in specific areas of endeavour rather than advocate a broad menu of actions that may only generate modest overall support. In the same vein, it may also be the case that some local governments may not wish to be tied down to a broad and ambitious approach by which they may be subsequently judged (particularly by the media) but rather take a more strategic and individualized approach to their social changes in this area of end of life care. In this way, the move towards a charter may be an outcome for some local governments rather than an opening ambit.

But whatever the precise approach to the adoption of the charter – now and for the future – our current feedback suggests that there is broad agreement within social and cultural organizations about some basic needs. Most local government/Mayoral offices agree that more can and should be done in end of life care than simply relying on services; that there is and can be a greater role for social and cultural organizations to play in addressing the gaps in service provision in end of life care; that policy development in the area of end of life care is particularly underdeveloped in the social (as opposed to clinical) sectors; and that it is often challenging to plan actions without a 'map' of where one should start to do things in the community that will maximize support outside of formal social and health service points. The charter provides a clear and simple sociological model of key institutions and events that are core to the life of most communities.

These points of agreement permit the creation of common ground from where all vested interests might begin a debate on the location and type of action areas where they wish to commence changes to their community that will enhance support at the end of life. This single key function of the charter invites social and cultural sectors into a practical discussion of what can, as well as what should, be done for their community. This is a practical call for implementation that has wide appeal and our current feedback suggests that this is crucial to engaging interest and commitment for these social and cultural sectors.

Conclusion

We continue to live in a time when there remains everywhere at best restraint (Appleby et al., 2014) and, at worse, modest increases against soaring costs (Deloitte, 2014) in funding for the public sector. In health and in social care provision we continue to look to do more with less or, at least, to be more effective with what resources remain to us. This has inadvertently breathed new life into public health initiatives that seek to mobilize alternative supports for the promotion of health, the prevention of illness, and the most expeditious methods for management of crisis, long-term care, and the triage and prioritization of urgent care. This is also true for all forms of end of life care – suicide and accident prevention, intensive care, care for frail older people, palliative care, bereavement care and dementia care. Rather ironically, as we confront these ongoing public sector challenges of diminishing resources we are also commonly confronted with a poverty of ideas about how to engage communities in helping us address these challenges.

As health service professionals, there remains a tendency to use what we know best – to employ volunteers, to initiate social marketing campaigns that preach to publics rather than engaging them, to make hospice the signature way to talk about death, dying or loss, or to speak about community engagement for specific disease groups (e.g. dementia). The Compassionate City Charter offers us a way forward and an opportunity to decentre our efforts away from a health services way of 'doing death and dying' and to break away from thinking about mortality in terms of specific diseases. The charter invites us to embrace two crucially important principles of our own health care and destiny. These are: (1) to ensure 'buy-in' from all sectors of the community by inviting the key social and cultural players to share the care; and (2) to remind all of us that death, dying, loss and caregiving is not more or less important because it occurs to the elderly or young children, because we have cancer or because we consider suicide, because I grieve for my stillborn child or you grieve for a lost dog. *All* dying, death, loss and caregiving experiences are important because each of these experiences diminish us in different but highly personal ways that can have detrimental health and social effects on us, our loved ones, those we work with, those we relax with, and those we pray with. And if quality of life in the modern world means facilitating and enhancing basic levels of health and wellbeing for everyone then the charter is one key way of creating a civic and dignified path to that goal in the face of our joint experiences of death and loss.

References

Appleby, J., Thompson, J. and Jabbal, J. (2014) How is the NHS performing? Quarterly monitoring report. London: King's Fund.

Deloitte (2014) *2014 Global Health Care Outlook: Shared Challenges, Shared Opportunities*. London: Deloitte Touche Tohmatsu.

Karapliagou, A. and Kellehear, A. (2014) *Public Health Approaches to End of Life Care: A Toolkit*. London: National Council for Palliative Care and Public Health England.

Kellehear, A. (1999) Health-promoting Palliative Care. Melbourne: Oxford University Press.

Kellehear, A. (2005) *Compassionate Cities: Public Health and End-of-Life Care*. London: Routledge.

Kellehear, A. (2009) Dying old – and *preferably* alone? Agency, resistance and dissent at the end of life. *International Journal of Ageing and Later Life* 4(1): 5–21.

Kumar, S. (2012) Public health approaches to palliative care: the Neighbourhood Network in Kerala. In: L. Sallnow, S. Kumar and A. Kellehear (eds) *International Perspectives on Public Health and Palliative Care*. Abingdon: Routledge, 98–109.

Sallnow, L., Kumar, S. and Kellehear, A. (eds) (2012) *International Perspectives on Public Health and Palliative Care*. Abingdon: Routledge.

7 'Join Bill United!'

Compassionate Communities in Limerick, Ireland

Kathleen McLoughlin and Jim Rhatigan

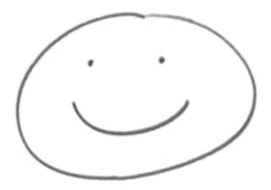

Figure 7.1 Photo of Bill
Source: Drawn by Rebecca Lloyd for the Milford Care Centre's Compassionate Communities Project (2011).

Once upon a time, there was a man called Bill.
He was living in Limerick City in his community of family, friends, neighbours, work colleagues and team mates.
One day, Bill went to see the doctor – his tests results were back.
The news wasn't good.
Incurable.

Bill is going to die.

He is devastated – so are his family.

Eventually Bill tells his world – his wife, his children, his family, his friends, his neighbours, his rugby pals. They are all shocked and sad, but all want to help him.
Bill's community are 'Bill United'.

'Bill United' harnesses Bill's care in his community bringing ideas, love, support and care together.

'Bill United' listens when Bill needs to talk.

When Bill is angry and when he is sad, they provide him with strength.

'Bill United' do what needs doing, to help Bill live in the best possible way.

Bill knows that 'Bill United' will support his family now ... and when he is gone.

Because Bill will die.

But he will die holding lots of hands, with the people he loves.

And 'Bill United'? They will go on to help others, creating a legacy that will go on ... and on ... and on ...

Bill's story is a simple story – a fairy tale perhaps? Are people like Bill, who are living with a serious illness and facing death, able to 'tell their world'? Does the community want to reach out and help? Do we, both as a society and as individuals, know what to say, what to do, when faced with issues of death, dying, loss and care – issues that are far from simple and yet will affect us all at some point in our life?

'Bill's Story' is a short animated film developed by Milford Care Centre's Compassionate Communities Project (Milford Care Centre, 2011). It represents what it means to live in, and be part of, a Compassionate Community. It serves as an important cornerstone to the project. It has had a worldwide audience, has been shown to an All-Party Committee in the UK House of Lords, and has been translated into Spanish and used extensively in Spain and South America, where Bill is known as 'Juan' (New Health Foundation, 2014). It is a story that provides both a vision for the project and serves as a tool to explain to people exactly what the Compassionate Communities concept is all about, in a way that engages people regardless of age, nationality or social background. Bill's Story is a gentle introduction to what is undoubtedly a hard subject.

Death, dying, loss and care in Ireland

Death, dying and loss are universal experiences. Every year in Ireland approximately 28,000 people die (Central Statistics Office, 2012), 80 per cent of whom die following a period of chronic illness (HSE, 2011). For every death that takes place it has been estimated that up to 10 other people are affected (Forum on End of Life, 2010) – that is potentially 280,000 people in Ireland every year. Most people who are living with advanced life-limiting illnesses spend their time at home and in their communities and neighbourhoods, with families, relatives, friends and work colleagues (HSE, 2011). The majority of people affected by advanced illness want to be cared for, and to die, at home (Weafer, 2014); however nationally, only one in four achieve that wish (McKeown, 2012).

Introducing Milford Care Centre

People like Bill, living in Limerick are usually familiar with Milford Care Centre, the specialist palliative care service for the Mid-West, providing care for individuals with advanced life-limiting illness. Milford is the first and only specialist palliative care provider in Ireland to make a strategic commitment to Health Promoting Palliative Care (HPPC) and is home to the country's only Compassionate Communities Project (CCP).

Fundamentally, a HPPC approach seeks to answer the question 'How do we use the experience and knowledge of the specialist palliative care service to support communities, groups and individuals to enhance the social, emotional and practical support available to those living with a life-threatening illness, those facing loss and those experiencing bereavement?' (McLoughlin et al., 2012). The approach combines specialist palliative care knowledge with health promotion methods and a community development philosophy. In taking a 'whole population' approach and by working in partnership with community organisations, groups and individuals the aim is to develop initiatives to prevent or minimise social difficulties, enhance capacities to cope and provide support to others in dealing, with issues of death, dying, loss and care (Kellehear, 1999, 2005). A helpful analogy to highlight the focus of HPPC is that of a river. It is an approach that distinguishes between the provision of services that are crucial when people are ill (downstream) and initiatives that focus on how issues of death, dying, loss and care are dealt with at a whole population/community level (upstream). HPPC seeks to influence what is happening 'downstream' and also to minimise harm from downstream factors (Rumbold and McInerney, 2012) by enhancing the capacity of individuals, groups and communities to cope with those experiences.

Milford Care Centre has a long history working in partnership with communities supporting them to live better with death, dying, loss and care through the social work team's commitment to community outreach in the bereavement service, through vibrant education projects and the multidisciplinary Hospice at Home service. Members of staff had performed a play, *Cancer Tales*, to a general public audience, film documentaries had been produced (e.g. Donnelly – *Going Home*) and research had been conducted in the broader applied aspects of death, dying, loss and care (e.g. Donnelly, 1999, 2010; McLoughlin, 2012).

The impetus for Milford to formally adopt a HPPC approach was underpinned by this tradition and a number of other important factors:

- Death, dying, loss and care affect everybody and are not just issues relevant to health and social care professionals.
- The experiences of death, dying, loss and care bring with them additional personal, health and social costs which are preventable and/or relievable if the right supports are available in the right place at the right time

(Kellehear, 2008; Wright et al., 2008; Dumont et al., 2006; Hebert et al., 2009).

- The majority of people living and eventually dying from advanced life-limiting illnesses spend the greater part of their time at home being cared for and supported by family members, friends and neighbours (HSE, 2011).
- Specialist palliative care services developed historically in response to the care needs of those affected by and dying from cancer. Between 80 per cent and 90 per cent of patients cared for by these services have a cancer diagnosis (DoH, 2001).
- The majority of people in Ireland do not die from cancer (CSO, 2012) and many have limited access to specialist palliative care services (HSE, 2011).
- Many people feel unprepared when faced with the experiences of advanced, life-limiting illnesses, death and bereavement and are uncertain as how to offer support and assistance.
- Specialist palliative care services have accumulated a wide range of skills, knowledge, expertise and information which are transferable to non-specialist settings, including the community and general public.

Milford Care Centre's Compassionate Communities Project

What is it like for those like Bill living with an advanced illness and facing death, who spend most of their last year of life at home, in their community with family and friends?

> I think we must look at the social context of dying in Ireland today. In Ireland death has been sanitised, put in the closet, so to speak. Until lately, speaking about death had almost become a taboo subject, resulting in a similar denial and fear of death that is prevalent throughout the Western World.
>
> (Carroll, 2010)

A lack of openness and the resulting low levels of public and professional awareness around issues relating to death and dying have implications for society as a whole and for people like Bill who are at the end of life (McLoughlin, 2012). In response to such concerns the Report of the Forum on End of Life in Ireland recommended a public health approach to end of life, emphasising that end of life issues are not just the responsibility of those who provide hospice and palliative care services, but require a response from society as a whole (Carroll, 2010). It is in this context that Milford Care Centre commenced the Compassionate Communities pilot project in January 2011 in a defined area of North West Limerick City. During this pilot, we listened to the issues for people living in the community (Brereton, 2012). Common themes included:

- The difficulty in talking about death, dying and bereavement (particularly to children).
- The experience that the emotional impact of loss is often unacknowledged.
- The cumulative and intense nature of the loss experienced by local communities particularly as a result of the number of young people who had died in tragic circumstances.

> She went up to the cemetery; she said every second grave at least was a young person. I suppose it's only when you look at the bigger picture because in some ways bereavement is a personal thing because it's just what happens around your circle. When you see all the circles and you see them together, it's shocking.

- The recognition of death as profound and mysterious, and the comfort and support found in religious faith and belief in an afterlife.
- Irish society was regarded as generally supportive of recently bereaved people. Ritual and remembrance of the dead were seen as important and as expressions of community solidarity for the bereaved.
- Concern that bereaved people are not always allowed sufficient time and space to grieve, and that sometimes social and practical support are withdrawn too soon.

> Often around death there is a huge fuss at the time and there is quite an intense kind of thing that goes on maybe for a few days or a week, but it is shocking then how much that is replaced by absolutely no intervention ... there was a massive fuss. But then that just absolutely evaporated and then there was nothing.

- Immediate family and friends were seen as the most important sources of support for people living with a life-limiting illness.

> Word of mouth, it would get around, And where people ... a lot of them went down and made sure his shopping was done ... That was people around, the neighbours actually did a lot, you know.

The listening exercise was a very important step in the process of engaging with the community and was used to frame potential responses to issues that emerged.

Following evaluation of the initial pilot (Brereton, 2012) the project was extended for a further 12 months, between June 2012 and May 2013, to the whole of Limerick City and to the rural town of Newcastlewest, thus providing two geographic areas diverse in both their location and population. Two part-time project workers were appointed, supported by a Project Operations Group, and managed by the principal social worker. This Phase 2 was also evaluated (McLoughlin, 2013). In April 2014, Milford committed to a three-year work plan, enabling the project to reach across the whole of the Mid-West.

The aims of the Compassionate Communities Project have remained consistent since 2011: 'To enrich and support society to live compassionately with death, dying, loss and care and to demonstrate and evaluate the process of developing a compassionate community model in an Irish context.'

The project has worked toward these aims by implementing a three-strand approach to its activities: a whole population approach; community engagement; a social model of care – the Good Neighbour Partnership (Figure 7.2). We have developed a formal 'Boiler Plate Statement' to summarise succinctly what the project is about:

> The experience of illness, dying and death affects all of us. But these things are never easy to deal with. Sometimes we aren't sure what we should say or what we should do. Talking about death and dying is difficult. We often don't know how we might help someone even when we want to. But not facing up to illness and loss as an important part of life only makes it harder for everyone. The Compassionate Communities Project is an initiative of Milford Care Centre. We are here to support people in the Mid-West to think a little differently about death, to

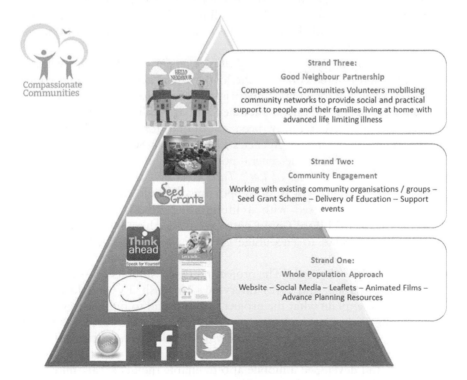

Figure 7.2 The Compassionate Communities Project model of activity

encourage people to plan ahead, talk with others and offer practical support within the community to those facing the end of life. A small change in our attitude toward death can make a big difference to how we live.

This statement is important as it allows a vision to be shared and clear messages developed as part of an agreed marketing plan. The work of the project is aligned to the three core strands of activity.

Strand One: a whole population approach

Our Compassionate Communities Project takes a whole population approach by:

- *Reaching out via the Internet through the project website and social media* The website (www.compassionatecommunities.ie) now has over 40,000 hits from more than 120 countries, with significant traffic from the UK and Ireland, Australia, New Zealand and America. Engagement via social media is steadily increasing (facebook.com/billunited and Twitter @CompassionateCP). Whilst there is little evidence that people are *publically* engaging on social media, we are aware of the impact posts have when, for example, we call for volunteers. This suggests that followers may read the posts, reflect on them *personally and act on them in specific circumstances.*
- *Development of a series of Let's Talk leaflets* (available on the website). Over 3,000 printed copies of the leaflets have been distributed widely throughout GP practices and primary care teams, universities and education sector, libraries, churches and at public and project events. The leaflets have recently been submitted for approval under the National Adult Literacy Agencies Plain English Scheme to ensure that they are accessible to the general population.
- *Development of a series of Let's Talk films* Five companion films have been produced as a way of supporting difficult conversations when someone is diagnosed with a life-limiting illness. The social work department in Milford Care Centre are using these films with patients and their families to encourage open discussion and exploration of issues.
- *Engaging with the media* The project regularly submits press releases to local newspapers and gives interviews on Irish TV and local radio stations to explain what the project is about and to publicise events.
- *Working with a local university to develop tools and resources for the project, e.g. short films and mobile apps* Graduates from the University of Limerick have written, directed and produced a short film for the project and developed a mobile app to enable the Let's Talk films to be displayed on mobile phones/tablets.

- *Engagement through public events* Staff from the University of Limerick, with support from their business connections, built a 'Before I Die' board that is used as a way of engaging people of all ages during public events, e.g. the Saturday market in the City. The board, standing more than eight feet tall, prompts people to start talking, ask questions, take leaflets and make connections.
- *Promoting Think Ahead* The Think Ahead initiative has been developed by the Irish Hospice Foundation's Forum on End of Life to encourage people to 'Think, Talk and Tell' regarding their wishes for end of life. It is a tool to guide members of the public in discussing and recording their preferences in the event of emergency, serious illness or death.

It's about making a human connection

On a Saturday in October 2014, the project went to Limerick's Milk Market with the 'Before I Die' board and a range of leaflets. A member of the public approached the project coordinator and explained that her dad was about to receive some 'bad news' about his health. She didn't know what to do, she was upset and became very emotional as she said 'He's my Dad, I just love him so much.' The project coordinator listened and took the time to engage with her, during which another member of the public came over to take a leaflet, explaining that her sister had died a few years ago. She started to engage with the woman whose father was unwell and offered words of support and advice. Five minutes later, the women decided *they would go and have a cup of coffee together.*

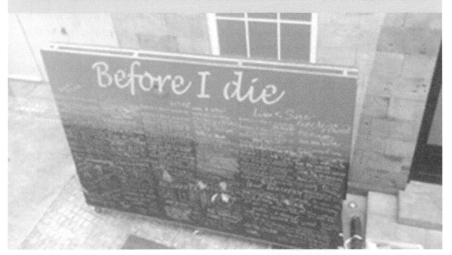

Figure 7.3 The 'Before I Die' board at Limerick Milk Market
Source: Photo by Kathleen McLoughlin.

Strand Two: community engagement

A core part of the Compassionate Communities project worker role is to identify and engage community organisations, statutory and voluntary groups in the geographical areas with the purpose and aims of the project. At a practical level, a mapping exercise is completed with each new phase of the project to determine the key agencies/groups within the catchment area. The impact of this approach can vary, depending on the region. For example in Phase 2 of the project, it was easier to network in Newcastlewest, a clearly defined area with a relatively small number of potential groups and partners. In contrast, Limerick City was described as 'vast ... a huge area' by the assigned project worker. The city is made up of diverse groups and there are so many organisations, that it can be difficult to work with the groups in an intense way: 'I feel like I am just out there scattering seeds thinly and hoping some of them take root.'

Community development work is a slow process and it can be difficult to demonstrate impact to funders (Lewis, 2006). Whilst networking can take time, it is a vital first step in engagement in the development of active relationships from a community partnership perspective. Where possible, it would be beneficial for the project worker to have a base in the region supported at low/no cost by one of the community agencies. This has the added benefit of raising the visibility of the project locally.

A west Limerick farmer was thinking ahead

We give out resources like Think Ahead, but we never know what happens as a result. It could take years to see and measure the impact of giving someone an advanced planning document at a public event. But we know that for at least one person it had made a powerful difference. We heard from a staff member working in an acute hospital that an elderly farmer, who had been admitted to hospital and who was dying, shared with her the fact that he 'had one of those forms'. She asked to see it and it was removed carefully from his bag, wrapped in newspapers and envelopes with two elasticated cables securing it carefully. In the form, the farmer described how he wanted to die at home, in his own bed. She asked him if she could share his form with the doctor. Initially he said no, explaining 'I don't want to undermine what he is doing' but eventually agreed and procedures were put in place to discharge the man, with home supports. The west Limerick farmer achieved his wish to die at home, on the farm.

The community engagement strand of the project plan is built around informing people of the purpose and aims of the project and engaging with them about the issues of death, dying, loss and care, using a variety of approaches. The plan calls for an approach that enables people to determine their own needs, partner with the project to address them and to support people/groups to take action. It is important that there are concrete tools/ resources and agreed methodologies to frame engagement, e.g. leaflets, seed grant scheme, education programmes. Over the course of the year in Phase 2 of the project in Limerick City and Newcastlewest, the fruits of the intensive collaboration are easy to see. At least 170 distinct contacts were made with agencies and groups across a diverse range of sectors including schools, higher and adult education providers, children and family community services, parishes, emergency and defence services, HSE services, sporting organisations, An Garda Síochána (the police), voluntary and community non-governmental organisations such as Le Chéile, Paul Partnership, the City Council, employment services, Lions Club, Macra, probation services, libraries, local politicians, potential high-profile champions and members of the general public. Whilst some of these contacts did not reach fruition, there was joint communication regarding roles and work programmes. For some this is where contact with the project ceased, following what appeared to be a high level of initial interest. One project worker said 'It's obvious after a few moments if someone is interested. They either get it or they don't.' Those reported to most likely 'get it' were those who had had a significant experience with death, dying, loss and care in their own life and could therefore relate the project to their personal/ professional experience. In some cases where the seeds of contact reached fruition the impact shows a clear trajectory of positive development. Examples of successful engagement during Phase 2 of the project include:

- A community arts group exhibition 'The Journey' on the theme of death, dying, loss and care.
- A county town hosting a community-led Ribbons of Remembrance service.
- Public talks by well-known speakers on grief and loss.
- A film club event on the challenges of living with and dying from Alzheimer's disease.
- A collection of poems on the theme of death, dying, loss and care written by students in a local secondary school.
- Morning briefing sessions at each of the Limerick City Garda stations to outline the aims of the Compassionate Community Project.
- Creation of the 'Before I Die' stand with volunteers from the departments of Engineering and Design, University of Limerick, and local businesses.
- Engagement with trainees in a probation service project to create a series of wooden memory bowls on behalf of Milford Hospice, from the Light up a Memory Tree.

Seed grant scheme

The aim of the seed grant scheme is to provide financial support to inspire and support community groups, organisations and individuals who wish to mark in some tangible way their response to the universal realities of death, dying, loss and care as experienced by those living, working or studying within their communities. Applications for the funding are encouraged from organisations, groups and individuals throughout the Mid-West. Since the project commenced, 15 seed grants have been awarded. The projects funded have been diverse in nature, developed by local organisations, in partnership with the local community, and are all relevant to the area of death, dying, loss and care. Examples include:

- *Local libraries* Permanent Compassionate Communities Bibliotherapy Resources available through the library.
- *Third level college* Development of mindfulness project to support staff and students who are having difficulty in coping with issues relating to death, dying and loss.
- *Children and family support service* Resources associated with death, dying, loss and care for use with children and families.
- *Local Family Resource Centre* Supporting the monthly drop-in grief and loss group and training of Community Ambassadors.
- *Rural support service* Two workshops re: supporting parents/children through bereavement.

It is clear from engagement with these organisations that had the seed grant scheme not been made available, these projects may never have reached fruition, or would have been delayed considerably. The range of organisations across Limerick and Newcastlewest engaging in this manner with the CCP and Milford Care Centre crosses many social boundaries – the general public, children and family services, higher education, the arts, older people's service and those with intellectual disabilities – bringing the work of the project to some of the most vulnerable groups in society. Historically, as a member of the Project Advisory Committee commented, 'these are groups that Milford Care Centre has never formally engaged with'. The projects developed are in the spirit of those discussed by Kellehear (2005) and the true value of these, when we consider the matched funding in the form of direct labour, time, additional donations, etc., is considerably more than the €8,665 invested. The positive social impact of such engagement and investment is clear when projects reach completion and the vast majority of the projects funded have produced sustainable outputs that will have an impact over many years beyond the completion of the work.

Case Study: Working with CARI – Children at Risk Ireland

Management at CARI contacted Milford Care Centre when a member of their team died from cancer. They wanted to know what support they could offer staff following her death. Through this contact, CARI learnt about the work of the Compassionate Communities Project and applied for a seed grant for a memorial garden in her honour that would also serve as a reflective space for staff and service users. The garden was opened in 2013 and they are now developing a bereavement policy and have the project resources on display.

Whilst the seed grant scheme is an area of interest in the project's liaison with community groups it was sometimes difficult for groups to see how the money could be utilised, particularly within the tight timeframes required for the grants awarded. Funding opportunities need to well advertised, through local press, community radio, via parish and school networks and online resources with regular calls for funding and deadlines so that people can plan their projects and applications well in advance. Consideration might also be given to making funding available for projects that may impact in any area of the Mid-West, regardless of the location of the person/group receiving the award. As the project momentum and communication mechanisms grow, it is envisaged that the scheme would operate without a need for the project to spend so much time supporting organisations to develop their ideas.

Education and training

'How I manage grief and loss' is a workshop, held over two half-days, made available in the community by the Compassionate Communities Project. This experiential workshop is aimed at people employed by community-based organisations or who have a role, within their working life, supporting people in their community affected by death, dying, loss and care issues. Participants attending would not have usually taken the learning and development opportunities offered by Milford Care Centre. Day One of the workshop includes warm up activities, individual and group reflection on personal experiences of loss and completion of a River of Life's Losses and reflection. Day Two focuses on understanding of grief, factors that may make grief additionally difficult and strategies for providing support.

The workshops evaluate very positively and have been demonstrated to reduce death anxiety and improve confidence in one teacher group who undertook the programme during their summer continuing professional development (CPD) programme. One participant reflected:

I had done training at Milford years ago, and I did the bereavement education years ago. I came to these workshops thinking I knew it all, I had heard it all before. But I was shocked at how much I learned and benefited from being there. The trainers are expert facilitators, wonderful. I couldn't believe when I did my River and compared it with the one I did years ago, how much I had had to deal with. When you work with vulnerable families, you lose that rawness. Being on that course has made me realize how strong I am and how raw those people really feel.

This valuable, but resource-intensive course requires advanced facilitation skills and the support of staff working in the social work and bereavement service. The project team continue to offer this programme twice a year but are currently exploring other programmes that can be delivered in a less resource-intensive way.

Café conversations

Café conversations for organisation-specific participants and the general public on issues related to death, dying, loss and care are organised in conjunction with community partners throughout the region. They present an opportunity for people to come together to talk about death, dying, loss and care in a community space. Approximately 100 people attended café conversations in Phase 2 of the project. One attendee described it as 'a lovely gentle introduction' to death, dying, loss and care, whilst another said: 'Public meetings work well, but the Café Conversations are hard, they need to be themed so people have a real focus, the general approach doesn't really work, people need to be guided.'

Working with schools

In Phase 1 of the pilot, the CCP explored the idea of initiating a death education programme in the primary school sector to provide support for children in dealing with the experience of death, dying, loss and care. However, some resistance was met from both parents and teachers. A focus group with representation from a cross-section of schools in the area felt that the term 'Death Education' was too stark, but agreed that information and support in the form of suitable literature and books for children would be well received and that grief and loss workshops with specific reference to the teaching profession would be beneficial to colleagues. It was also recommended that the optimum way to proceed was for the project to visit schools individually and explore their needs.

Visiting individual schools is time-consuming and despite some positive engagement the general reaction was mixed. Consequently a decision was then taken to adopt a more strategic approach and a regional group of key leaders and partners in the education sector was established to develop engagement with schools. Work is currently underway to develop a directory of supports for teachers, proposals are being developed to establish a CPD programme for teachers and to consider the potential for the designation of Compassionate Schools.

Community engagement – challenges

Contact with a wide range of organisations and agencies during the 12-month period of Phase 2 of the project led to very positive developments. However, community engagement at this level is time-consuming, labour-intensive work and questions of capacity and sustainability have to be addressed. In particular, the dilemma for the CCP is whether it should continue engaging directly with as broad a range of community organisations as possible, or whether it would be more effective to join with a small number of community partners in defined locations and to plan a series of targeted events in areas throughout the Mid-West. This more focused approach, together with a strong media/PR plan, aimed at the general public, would promote change and action within the community. As one member of the public attending a Compassionate Communities event commented: 'if we could just get four practical talks a year on this topic with a good attendance of 50 people at each one, we'd be making a real difference'.

An aim of the project is 'To enrich and support society to live compassionately with death, dying, loss and care'; it is clear that there is considerable work required to raise awareness of the importance of this field and encourage people to become confident in talking about these issues, before they can ever be expected to do things differently. This in turn supports the need to focus on enabling thought and conversation and having a clear call to action, within which to engage people in the community.

Strand Three: a social model of care – the Good Neighbour Partnership

We would all like to live in an area where people look out for and help each other. This creates a sense of belonging for those who receive the support and it also gives those who help a sense of purpose as they 'give something back' to their community. For people like Bill, living with a serious illness can be difficult. It can be hard to do the ordinary everyday things when you have to cope with not feeling well, or think about doctors' appointments, go to and from hospital or juggle the demands of caring. Often friends and neighbours want to help, but are sometime unsure how to. The project, together with community organisations, is developing a model of volunteer-led, free social and practical support to people living at home, with advanced life-limiting illness. The aims of the Good Neighbour Partnership are:

• To enable people living with palliative care needs in the community to identify their social and practical needs.

- To enable the social and practical needs to be met from within the person's circle of community.

In fulfilling these aims, it is anticipated that there may be an impact on a person's quality of life, psychosocial wellbeing and unplanned health service use. In addition, such a model may reduce carer burden and build community capacity to engage in issues associated with death, dying, loss and care. We envisage that this strand of the project is the key to moving Bill's Story from an aspiration to a reality. Over the next two years, with funding from the All Ireland Institute of Hospice and Palliative Care, Irish Cancer Society, Irish Hospice Foundation and Milford Care Centre, the proposed model will be further developed and evaluated using the Medical Research Council (MRC) Framework for Complex Interventions (McLoughlin et al., 2014). Fifteen volunteers have already been recruited with almost equal numbers of men and women expressing interest in delivering the model of support. We anticipate that support to people living at home will commence in early 2015.

The future

Milford Care Centre's Compassionate Communities Project now spans across the whole of the Mid-West, guided by a comprehensive plan with a three-year time frame. Goals for the future include enabling Limerick to fulfil the Compassionate City Charter (Kellehear, 2014) and to become the first Compassionate City in Ireland. It is vital to ensure that everything we do is evaluated, both in terms of process and impact. We know that 58 per cent of people in the Mid-West have heard about the project (Weafer, 2014) and that those who are more familiar with the project are more likely to have taken positive action regarding planning for end of life (Weafer, 2014). These statistics provide a baseline that we hope will increase further over the next phase of our work. Such statistics are important to funders and planners.

Our work is receiving national recognition. For example, the project was referred to in Seanad Eireann during a motion on developing an end of life and bereavement strategy for Ireland. Senator O'Donnell (2014) said:

> In other areas citizens have taken brilliant initiatives such as the Compassionate Communities project at Milford Care Centre in Limerick which seeks to work in partnership with individuals, groups and communities facing loss and those experiencing bereavement.
>
> The State must learn from these initiatives and catch up with community-led creative solutions. We need the panoply of State services to help us to think, talk and tell about dying, death and loss and enable us to support each other.

Such recognition reignites the passion and commitment of the project team and Milford Care Centre to strive toward our aims and objectives. We want to be able to ensure that people like Bill, who want to talk about end of life, have the vocabulary, skills and resources to do so. We want Bill's community to have the vocabulary, skills and resources to help. We want people to feel empowered and know what to say and what to do, when faced with issues of death, dying, loss and care.

Our future looks toward supporting people like Bill and Bill United and in doing so creating a legacy that will go on ... and on ... and on ...

Acknowledgements

With sincere thanks to Marie Richardson, Principal Social Worker, who worked with communities in North West Limerick in the first phase of the project (2010–11) and who continues as an active member of the Project Operation Group. Mary Brereton who conducted the evaluation of the first phase of the project and Rebecca Lloyd who has been a special contributor to the project through the development of 'Bill's Story' and 'Let's Talk' film series. Carmelita McGloughlin and Caroline Macken, project workers during Phase 2 of the project and of course a warm thank you to everyone who has shared their stories, time and memories with us since we started our journey.

References

Brereton, M. (2012) *Report on the Evaluation of Milford Care Centre's Compassionate Communities Project*. Limerick: Milford Care Centre.Carroll, B. (2010) *Report of Forum on End of Life*. Dublin: Irish Hospice Foundation.

Central Statistics Office (2012) *Vital Statistics: Four Quarter and Yearly Summary*. Dublin: CSO. www.cso.ie/en/media/csoie/releasespublications/documents/vital stats/2012/vstats_q42012.pdf

Department of Health and Children (2001) *Report of the National Advisory Committee on Palliative Care*. Dublin: Department of Health and Children.

Donnelly, S. (1999) Folklore associated with dying in the West of Ireland. *Palliative Medicine* 13(1): 57–62.

Donnelly, S. (2010) Relatives experience of the moment of death in a tertiary referral hospital. *Mortality* 15(1): 81–100.

Dumont, S., Turgeon, J., Allard, P., Gagnon, P., Charbonneau, C. and Vezina, L. (2006) Caring for a loved one with advanced cancer: determinants of psychological distress in family caregivers. *Journal of Palliative Medicine* 9(4): 912–921.

Forum on the End of Life in Ireland (2010) *Perspectives on End of Life – Report of the Forum 2009*. Dublin: Irish Hospice Foundation.

Health Service Executive (HSE) (2011) *Primary Palliative Care in Ireland*. Dublin: Irish Hospice Foundation.

Hebert, R., Schulz, R., Copeland, V. and Arnold, R. (2009) Preparing family caregivers for death and bereavement. Insights from caregivers of terminally ill patients. *Journal of Pain and Symptom Management* 37(1): 3–12.

Kellehear, A. (1999) *Health Promoting Palliative Care*. Melbourne: Oxford University Press.

Kellehear, A. (2005) *Compassionate Cities: Public Health and End-of-Life Care*. London: Routledge.

Kellehear, A. (2008) Health promotion and palliative care. In: Mitchell, G. (ed.) *Palliative Care: A Patient Centred Approach*. Oxford: Radcliffe.

Lewis, H. (2006) *New Trends in Community Development*. L/Derry: INCORE.

McKeown, K. (2012) *Place of Death in Ireland*. Dublin: Irish Hospice Foundation.

McLoughlin, K. (2012) Identifying and changing attitudes toward palliative care: an exploratory study. Unpublished doctoral thesis, Maynooth University, Ireland.

McLoughlin, K. (2013) *Evaluation of Milford Care Centre's Compassionate Communities Project*. Limerick: Milford Care Centre.

McLoughlin, K., Rhatigan, J. and Richardson, M. (2012) *Compassionate Communities Phase Two Project Plan, June 2012 to May 2013*. Limerick: Milford Care Centre.

McLoughlin, K., Rhatigan, J., Kellehear, A., McGilloway, S., Lucey, M., Twomey, F., et al. (2014) *Exploratory delayed intervention randomised controlled trial to assess the feasibility, acceptability and potential effectiveness of a volunteer-led model of social and practical support with community dwelling adults living with advanced life-limiting illness: Study Protocol*. (Prepared for submission).

Milford Care Centre (2011) *Bill's Story* (The original). www.youtube.com/watch?v=mqYmTTY-3gs

New Health Foundation (2014) *La historia du Juan*. www.youtube.com/watch?v=ugri9Q3oXQg

Rumbold, B. and McInerney, F. (2012) *A Public Health Palliative Approach*. Palliative Care Unit, School of Public Health, La Trobe University, Melbourne. www.palliativecare.org.au/Portals/46/APCC/Presentations/RUMBOLD_Bruce_PRSENTATION.pdf (Accessed 31 May 2012).

Weafer, J.A. (2014) *Irish Attitudes to Death, Dying and Bereavement 2004–2014*. Dublin: Irish Hospice Foundation.

Wright, A.A., Zhang, B., Ray, A., Mack, J.W., Trice, E., Balboni, T., et al. (2008) Associations between end-of-life discussions, patient mental health, medical care near death, and caregiver bereavement adjustment. *Journal of the American Medical Association* 300(14): 1665–1673.

8 Caring community in living and dying in Landeck, Tyrol, Austria

Klaus Wegleitner, Patrick Schuchter and Sonja Prieth

> Death is a fateful moment for social cohesion. It may rupture relationships among the living, it may reveal or generate extreme isolation, it may create a temporary community, or it may foster new and enduring relationships.
>
> (Walter, 1999: 123)

Building compassionate communities to promote caring democracy and 'caring society'

The question of a 'good life' and handling existential vulnerability and uncertainty

When we are confronted with life-limiting illness, vulnerability, dying, death and loss, our life plans, our feelings of security and our human existence are shaken to the core. The fragility of life becomes clear. In the interviews we have conducted, family carers have described this existential situation through various expressions, such as 'the collapse of a world'. These fragile personal life-worlds are embedded in late modern or, according to Zygmunt Bauman (2000), 'liquid' modern societies. In principle, we live and die under conditions of constant uncertainty. Modern biographies are more and more fractured and social networks and relationships have become increasingly tenuous. Current political and social developments in Europe – for example the rise of social injustice across Europe, youth unemployment, crises in elderly care, inhumane refugee policies, warlike events in Ukraine and at the borders of Turkey – all threaten social peace. We are facing apparently insoluble social, ethical and ecological problems on a global scale, as side effects of industrial modernity. In a confusingly complex world, there is a great need for security and social cohesion. However, most international and global policy responses to these problems have largely failed, or have revealed political helplessness.

Industrial modernity yields socially, technologically, economically and ecologically negative effects. This has evoked a set of different counter-movements in various social spheres since the middle of the twentieth century. Global health problems have led to the emergence of public health and health promotion (World Health Organization (WHO), 1978, 1986), global environmental problems to the sociopolitical discourse of sustainable development (WCED, 1987; Brundtland 1989) and to the ecological movement. The social taboo of death and dying, the inhumane conditions in hospitals as places in which to die and the therapeutic approaches of a paternalistic, exclusively biomedically oriented modern medicine (Saunders, 2000; WHO, 1990) all result from the 'industrialization of health care'. The modern hospice movement and transitions in end-of-life care can be understood as a reaction to these social developments. Fundamentally, the hospice movement, health promotion and sustainable development all have one thing in common: they raise the question of 'a good life', for all, in all phases of life, globally and also for future generations. In hospice care a good life includes death and dying; it therefore is a good life to the end. These movements and policies represent attempts to deal with the existential vulnerability and uncertainty of human life and of nature. In the respective strategies personal life-world and lifestyle interact with living, dying and caring conditions, with settings and sociopolitical frameworks.

In times of serious social challenges, uncertainties and upheavals, communities have become places in which people hope and yearn to find social warmth and security, perhaps even in a romanticized way (Bauman, 2001). Communities have also been established as places and spheres of social transition and change. The community ideally represents a social fabric in which public, political and ethical discourses take place, civil society is engaged, relationships, solidarities and networks are strengthened, support is organized, empowerment is promoted and caring responsibilities are distributed and assumed. The Healthy Cities Programme driven by health promotion and the Local Agenda 21 programme driven by sustainable development have both demonstrated the potential of community engagement and participation in the implementation of sociopolitical strategies (Hancock, 1997; Dooris, 1999). Building up 'community capital' is therefore described as the precondition and challenge in terms of developing healthy and sustainable communities in the twenty-first century (Hancock, 2001). In hospice and end-of-life care, the awareness of the social importance of community development and capacity building has also increased significantly over the last decade (Sallnow and Paul, 2014).

Caring democracy and sustainable development

According to the feminist political philosopher Joan Tronto, the answer to the question of 'a good life' involves caring in a broad and fundamental sense: 'caring … *includes everything that we do to maintain, continue, and repair our "world" so that we can live in it as well as possible. That world includes our bodies, our selves, and our environment*' (Fisher and Tronto, in Tronto, 2013: 19; original emphasis). Tronto's ethics of care raises fundamental questions: How can caring responsibilities be distributed in societies? How can they be assigned democratically (consistent with justice, equality and freedom)? How can we ensure the greatest possible participation of citizens in this assignment of responsibilities? These questions should be placed at the centre of democratic politics. Hence, the extent to which a caring democracy and a solidarity-oriented caring culture in society is realized and promoted indicates the degree to which a society's political system is democratic as a whole (Tronto, 2013).

Sustainable development ensures the future viability of our societies by balancing economic, social and environmental dimensions and responsibilities. Questions of how societies organize and enable care, solidarity and social participation address key aspects of sustainability (WCED, 1987). For example, in order to establish sustainable care for the dying and their relatives, the amount and location of economic and human resources invested by health policy are crucial. It makes a difference whether money is spent for acute medicine or for long-term care, whether it is invested in professional service-oriented care or in community-based care, in organizational structures or in social processes in communities. The latter opens a space in which compassion, as an ethical imperative for health (Kellehear, 2005: 44), and solidarity could arise. These decisions are social, political and ethical at the same time; they relate to sustainability and they are highly emotionally charged.

Compassion and sustainable care

With regard to death, loss and caring for the dying, the importance of community has been discussed in manifold ways (Walter, 1999; Maddocks, 2003; Kellehear, 2005; Dörner, 2007), and different models of community engagement have been illustrated and analysed (e.g. Kellehear, 2005; Sallnow and Paul, 2014; Barry and Patel, 2013).

It seems to us that the following three interpretations are connected with each other. All are of particular importance: First, introduced by Tony Walter (1999), *'death provides a basis for relationships and community'*. This means that shared, existential and universal experiences of death and loss foster social cohesion and generate a sense of community. Second, *'the community is a partner in end-of-life care'*, which is best represented through the first projects of health promoting palliative care in Australia (Kellehear, 1999, Rumbold, 2012). Recognizing and facing the limits of direct professional service provision in end-of-life care, palliative care services have built community partnerships. Third, *'care for the dying by the community'*, is central to the vision of the *compassionate community* movement (Kellehear, 2005) as well as the concept of a *caring culture in the third social space* (Dörner, 2007). In its most empowered form, this is characterized by broad civic engagement in everyday life within the wider community, in which members take on care responsibilities and control of care practices (Sallnow and Paul, 2014).

The compassionate community is an expression of shared values and fundamental ethical attitudes, such as empathy, mindfulness, attentiveness, respect and solidarity in human coexistence. Developing compassionate communities can be understood as a continuous cultural development process which enables immediate concern for vulnerable, frail, dying and bereaved people. These shared existential human experiences strengthen social resources and social cohesion, and promote supportive experiences and environments. Martha Nussbaum contextualizes compassion in public culture as a political conception 'that attempts to win an *overlapping consensus* among citizens of many different kinds, respecting the spaces within which they each elaborate and pursue their different reasonable conceptions of the good' (Nussbaum, 2003: 401). This requires spaces and opportunities in the community for ethical reflection of 'the good' in living and dying, in the interaction between individual and collective experiences, ideas and concepts; in the sense of a practising ethics (see Schuchter and Heller, Chapter 9 in this volume). According to this, community development processes that address the questions of how we want to live and to die in the future and how we could care for each other in a compassionate and democratic way are matters of society's sustainable development in its core meaning. With this in mind, evolving compassionate communities make an important contribution to 'care for our world', and therefore to a sustainable and 'caring society'.

A paradigmatic shift from service-centred end-of-life care to community care – the Austrian situation

The hospice and palliative care movement has developed considerably, especially over the last two decades. This is the case in Austria (Pelttari et al., 2014) as well as internationally (Centeno et al., 2013). As our societies struggle to enable human and compassionate end-of-life care for 'all who need it', the European Union's health care policy (Council of Europe – European Health Committee, 2003) has also taken into account the growing importance of palliative care. Therefore integrating palliative care into national healthcare systems has been a political priority for more than 10 years. In Austria, a political framework for the implementation of palliative care has been launched, with the title of '*Abgestufter Hospiz- und Palliativplan*' ('Graded hospice – and palliative care plan'). The plan was developed by a national panel of experts (Nemeth and Rottenhofer, 2004) having gained international recognition in the European palliative care community (European Association for Palliative Care (EAPC), 2009). These efforts have led for the most part to establishing specialist palliative care services – such as palliative care units, specialist palliative care teams, hospices and hospice teams. At the same time, increasing attention has been paid throughout Europe to professionalization, standardization and routinization (Centeno et al., 2013; EAPC, 2009).

Thus development in hospice and palliative care in Austria and in German-speaking Europe is focused on improving professional practice and specialized services, building up 'professionalized' volunteer services and developing organizations of 'dying experts'. This gives rise to fundamental social challenges: While palliative care services and structures are increasingly optimized death and dying are delegated to organizations and experts. This rather contributes to than mitigates the problem that many people have increasingly lost confidence in their own capacities, skills and self-help resources when confronted with vulnerability, life-limiting illness, suffering, dying and loss. Familiarity with local traditions and rituals of farewell has also gradually declined. Finally, the original idea of the hospice movement, to reintegrate death into everyday living patterns and to make dying and loss normal valued parts of life, cannot be promoted in this way.

When we acknowledge that end-of-life care is everyone's responsibility (Kellehear, 2013), then we as a society cannot delegate dying, death and loss to our modern care organizations, nor should this be pushed back into private spheres, which would still mean that it would rest on the shoulders of womankind. We have to create new (or rediscover old) forms of solidarity and compassion in the 'third social space' (Dörner, 2007) between private households and institutionally provided care; in the neighbourhood, in the district, in the diverse living spheres of community. Therefore, civil society's caring culture in all phases of life needs to be strengthened and the sovereignty of concerned people over their living and dying in their respective settings and life-worlds, 'where people live, love and work', to be encouraged, as already outlined in principle in WHO's report on primary health care (WHO, 1978) and in the Ottawa charter for health promotion (WHO, 1986). Inspired by developments in community-based palliative care in Kerala (Kumar, 2007) and in health promoting palliative care in Australia (Kellehear, 1999; Rosenberg and Yates, 2010), many encouraging models and projects all over the world (Sallnow et al., 2012) have emerged to address these public health concerns in end-of-life care.

Against this background, and building on its own tradition of health promoting palliative care in organizations and regional networks (Heller, 1996; Heimerl and Wegleitner, 2013), the Institute of Palliative Care and Organizational Ethics/Faculty of Interdisciplinary Studies (IFF Vienna) has developed a research programme called 'promoting communal care culture at the end-of-life', to foster the paradigmatic shift from professional- and institution-centred end-of-life care to community-based approaches in current palliative and dementia care.

Caring community in Landeck: the model project

In the following section, we describe the project 'Caring community in living and dying' in the Tyrolean community Landeck. It aims to strengthen networks and solidarity in the community in order to support older people in everyday life and family caregivers, furthermore to improve the local relationship between formal and informal caregivers in end-of-life care. The project follows community-based participatory research (Minkler and Wallerstein, 2003; Hockley et al., 2013) and a community development approach (Kellehear, 2005). The process should raise awareness within the local population about existential questions concerning vulnerability, frailty, dying, death, loss and grief, and about questions of 'caring democracy' (Tronto, 2013), prevention and caring networks. Self-help resources should be fostered and local initiatives and projects in diverse community contexts should be developed and supported. A collective process of developing a care culture in the everyday life of the community should be promoted. As this is an ongoing project, which began in 2013 and will finish at the end of 2015, we give an overview of developments to date, describing and reflecting on the project processes and interpreting the preliminary results.

Establishing the project structure: listening to each other and acting in partnership

The project was not initially launched by an organization or provider of hospice and palliative care and it was not a response to the directly articulated or perceived needs of a certain community. It began as a research and development concern of the IFF Vienna as a university and research institute and was conceived as an answer to the lack of community involvement in end-of-life care in Austria. It was clear from the very beginning that such a project thrives on the fruitful interaction between theory and practice. Therefore we enhanced the existing partnership with the Tyrolean Hospice Association, which operates on the one hand as a practice partner and on the other hand as a genuine research partner in terms of concrete cooperation in the research team. The project philosophy and an approximate project design were drawn up jointly. We then 'searched' for a suitable community for 'our' pilot project, and finally established a project partnership with local officials for social affairs and the municipality of Landeck, a district capital with 8,000 inhabitants situated in the rural mountain region of western Tyrol in Austria. Community representatives gave their trust to the project team and so a series of public events, interviews, focus groups, workshops and meetings could start in the name of the community, which gave momentum to the project.

'Why was Landeck chosen for the project?' This question was asked at some stage by interview partners, local stakeholders, the mayor and municipal councillors, indeed by virtually everybody with whom we had contact throughout the project. They felt honoured on the one hand but appeared concerned on the other, asking 'Is the situation in our region worse than it is in other regions of Austria?'

It is not the subject of the project to compare regions and their caring cultures, nor to assess or rate the quality of caregiving and care-receiving in a certain region. We wanted to facilitate the creation of a caring community in dying, which is not centred on specialized palliative care and is carried by civic society and primary health care. The area of Landeck was chosen as an example of an Austrian region where there are no specialized palliative care services (except coordinated hospice volunteers) and with long-established structures of civil society initiatives and a high level of civic commitment. Already prior to the project the informal care network in Landeck consisted of many people who provide various kinds of care for their nearest and dearest. Many inhabitants of Landeck offer their voluntary support (hospice group, self-care groups, family caregiver group, parish community, etc.) to people in the community who are either ill and frail or who are exhausted from the very challenging task of familial long-term care in which they live and work over many years. The formal care network includes a hospital in the neighbouring community of Zams, one nursing home in Landeck and two others nearby, a primary home care team, a private 24-hour home care service, together with domestic help services, and of course family doctors, who in many cases have known their elderly and frail patients for many years.

Thus each community has its own very specific existing caring networks, and a regionally developed caring culture. In beginning a compassionate community process through participatory research, the most important task is to make contact with people and to get a sense of the living conditions, the relationships, the caring spaces and places there; at the heart of this lies appreciating the existing situation and culture, coming together in conversation, listening and establishing mutual trust.

Participation, networking and shaping the future: the project design

The entire course of the project can be divided roughly into three phases.

Phase 1: Describing, analysing and appreciating local care cultures

- Building up content-related and social commitment in the community.
- Describing, analysing and appreciating local care cultures and traditions in end-of-life care within the framework of participatory research.
- Illustrating local care networks and resources, as well as self-help resources in end-of-life care.
- Nurturing a common understanding of care.

Phase 2: Strengthening local networks and self-help resources

- Strengthening networking between informal and formal care networks.
- Developing future perspectives of a caring community with wide participation.
- Developing local initiatives, mini-projects and measurements in various spheres of the community.

Phase 3: Supporting implementation and sustainability
- Supervising and supporting the implementation of initiatives and measures for caring networks in living and dying.
- Developing strategies of sustainability with local care team, steering committee and general public.

The project process enables the inhabitants of Landeck to exchange their experiences, to generate common knowledge of local care cultures and resources, and to engage in change at different system levels and in various spheres of the community (Figure 8.1). For example several settings for public discussion (citizenship forum, public future workshop, etc.) as well as local initiatives and interventions (public 'last aid' course, school project, caretaker/minder in the community, etc.) facilitate a broad involvement from concerned persons, citizens, (hospice) volunteers, healthcare professionals and providers, undertakers, pupils and teachers, self-help groups, the parish, representatives of clubs and associations and local politicians.

Phase 1: Describing, analysing and appreciating local care cultures

During our research we understood a caring community as 'networks of care relationships', which represent and offer 'realities of daily support' for the person concerned (Kellehear, 2005) through the interplay of 'circles of care' (Abel et al., 2013): starting with caring family members and friends as an inner network, through to less close family members, friends and neighbours as an outer network, the social capital or help resources of the

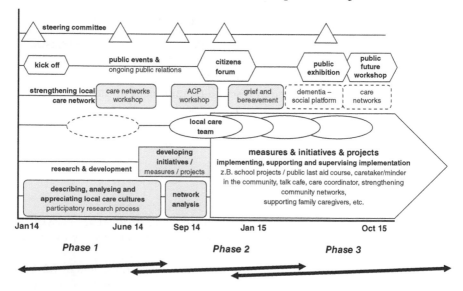

Figure 8.1 Project architecture and process

community, professional healthcare services, and up to the policy level as the outermost circle. We therefore began with focus groups comprising family caregivers, followed by focus groups and interviews with volunteers, then interviews and focus groups with professional caregivers and, finally, we conducted a workshop with informal and formal caregivers. After each enquiry setting, we conducted interim analyses to integrate these results into the design of the next research step and to feed it back twice – first at the steering committee level and then into local policy. In so doing, we based our research and intervention process on the dense narratives, micro-stories and care actions of people concerned in order to put these in relation to, and expand them with the different perspectives of, the 'circles of care'. We were not only collecting and analysing data but also initiating communication and fostering a growing awareness about both the needs of people at the end of their lives and the situation of those who care for them. Thus experiences and knowledge were already shared during the research process (Figure 8.2).

The following questions were of interest: How do people involved experience their living and caring situation? What kind of care, help and support do they need? What enables them to welcome and accept help? How could informal and formal care networks be strengthened? How could self-help resources of the community, of citizens, be encouraged? How is the relationship between informal and formal care networks organized? How could information about the diversity of care resources reach all those in

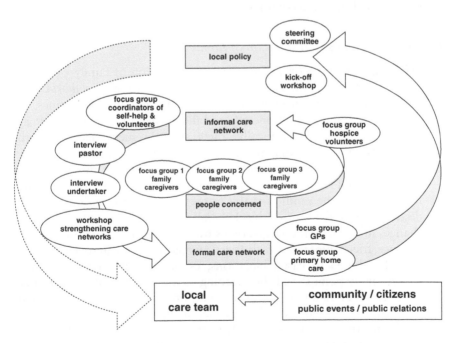

Figure 8.2 Sharing experiences and knowledge through participatory research

need and become common knowledge? How can we succeed in tackling the issues of vulnerability, dying, death, loss and grief at an early stage? How can we as a community prevent the social isolation and existential distress of family caregivers? How can we as a community begin a conversation about dying, death, loss and grief?

Some brief insights into the project process and contents of Phase 1

Focus groups with caring relatives

Generally speaking, we received positive responses to our interview requests, although carers encountered some difficulties in organizing the actual participation. It was obviously very challenging for them to leave the dependent relatives alone for a couple of hours or find somebody to look after them. We found a clear difference between women (since we had no information about any men being the main carers, we only talked to women) who were used to exchanging experiences and views with other caring relatives as members of a self-help group and those who were not. Statements like 'This is the first time I've ever told somebody about this' or 'I can't tell anybody because people don't want to know' show that primary carers tend to cope with the strain and pressure all by themselves. Especially where this second group of carers is concerned, conducting group interviews proved to be a positive intervention – carers began talking to one another and felt that finding they had things in common was beneficial.

The existential and social situation of family carers

- *'The collapse of a world'* The existential situation of family carers has been described in various expressions as the *collapse of a world*. This means that the familiar experience of everyday life and its routines, the familiar understanding of oneself, and the normal orientation in life are profoundly disturbed. Typically, there are two such collapses in the course of caring. First, and often gradually progressing, this takes place in the transition from 'normal' life to a life with permanent and demanding caregiving, and second, and more abruptly, with the death of the person receiving care (the mother or the father). The later situation has been described as 'falling into a black hole'. Both collapses entail dramatic changes in social relationships, one's own social role and self-image. For instance, friendships may break apart, and participation in social activities be reduced due to care obligations; essentially, questions are raised concerning happiness and the meaning of life: 'Is that all?' one woman said, or: 'What about my life?' Caring for others is experienced as a crisis that requires a fundamental reorientation in life, even for those who emphasize that it is natural to them to take on the role of the caring relative and that they experience it as a rewarding task.

- *The narrowness of caring* Nursing and caring in family situations is described as a burden that requires relief. Our findings and interpretations indicate that in addition to the burden of care work, the situation of family carers is marked by a specific quality which has been articulated in different terms expressing a certain 'narrowness' of caring. This narrowness starts with social isolation, but a distressing constriction of thinking and perception is also implied. The focus of attention is placed firmly on the person receiving care and the things that have to be done to fulfil his or her needs.
- *Guilt* A major and particularly difficult issue for family carers involves actual or potential feelings of guilt – the feeling of having done things wrong or thinking about transferring their cared-for relative to a nursing home. They feel highly obliged to do it all alone in best quality and meet the patient's desires really well.

Important 'ingredients' *of a compassionate community*

It became clear that not only experience, know-how and strengthening networks – the obvious aspects of organizing care – define care culture, as must be emphasized, when the human capacities to act are confronted with life's finiteness, there already exists 'wisdom', a form of indigenous knowledge, within the community. It also became apparent what the important 'ingredients' of *practical wisdom* around death and dying actually are. These insights should become shared knowledge and culture in the community through various project initiatives.

- *Experience of life* Persons 'who have seen a lot' or, even more so, persons who have themselves endured a period of illness or caring are particularly valuable to others. This is not because they can immediately give practical advice, but because they are considered as conversation partners who have the ability to *understand* someone who, for example, has to care for his mother or her father at home.
- *Keeping each other in mind/knowing about each other* This issue emerged when thinking about the role of neighbours in care situations and it revealed an ambiguity that is difficult to balance. On the one hand, a caring culture implies a living neighbourhood in such a way that people keep each other in mind and know about one another. A 'good' neighbour knows when somebody is not doing well and assists with small gestures of help. On the other hand, knowing about one another might quickly turn into some form of social control and gossip. Thus, the great art of caring between neighbours consists in people knowing about each other but without constricting each other's freedom and intimacy, and without producing false beliefs or confusing feelings of 'guilt'.

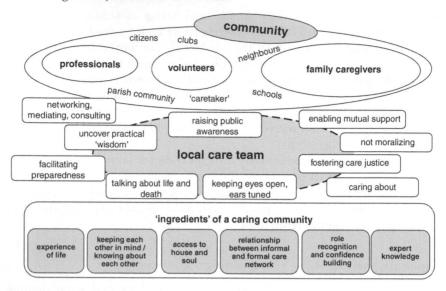

Figure 8.3 'Ingredients' of a caring community in Landeck

• *Access to house and soul* Being dependent on others and having to accept help from others can be experienced as humiliating or shameful. It is difficult to 'let others in' – both into one's 'soul' and life as well as into one's home. A compassionate community promotes a multifaceted art of caring that offers help in such a manner that persons in need find it easy (or easier) to *grant* access to house and soul.

• *Know-how in the sense of expert knowledge* is obviously what distinguishes healthcare professionals. However, family carers have often learned how to deal with catheters, suction systems or how to avoid the side-effects of drugs. In some cases, they have attended training courses in nursing techniques. Vice versa, expert know-how alone is not sufficient to enable healthcare professionals to be able to take care for others in a comprehensive sense of the word. The way in which a family doctor expressed this was: 'You need professional competence and a deeply human commitment.'

Based on the interviews, focus groups and workshops, Figure 8.3 gives an overview of the 'ingredients' and qualities that constitute a caring community.

Supporting and developing local initiatives

At the time of writing (October, 2014), we are midway through the decisive phase of the overall project. As a response to the intensive communication and coordination process within the action research project the stakeholders succeeded in building relationships of trust and in forming various 'care culture working groups' as parts of the 'local care team', which are particularly enthusiastic about a specific 'care initiative'.

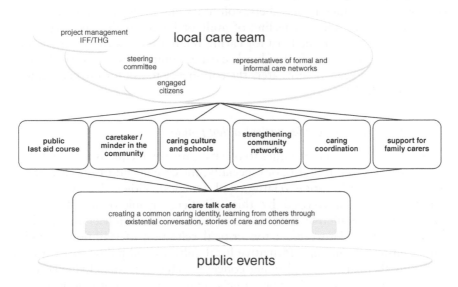

Figure 8.4 Local initiatives to make a caring community a reality in Landeck

The initiatives that have been launched cover different concerns and needs that have arisen during the research process, and represent the result of discussions in the steering committee (Figure 8.4). On the one hand, the initiatives aim at strengthening community members' self-help resources, raising public awareness and providing knowledge about issues regarding care, dementia, dying, death and loss (e.g. public 'last aid' course, different school and care culture projects and public events), as well as stimulating everyday solidarity and care for elderly persons living in single households. Regarding the latter, a 'caretaker in the community' project has been started and calls on professionals who at first glance are not identified with care for the elderly – e.g. hairdressers, postmen and women, the police, salespersons, etc. – to appreciate their role in everyday caring, to share care experiences and concerns, to strengthen their capacities in communicating with old and frail people and to develop specific strategies of caring for the elderly in conjunction with everyday working life. On the other hand, the initiatives should seek to improve the integration of local informal and formal caring networks (e.g. 'care networks workshops' and 'caring coordination') and to support caring relatives through end-of-life care.

Lessons learned

Creating viable care arrangements is a challenging task

There is a need to resolve or clarify issues such as securing a broad consensus in society that familial care is an extremely challenging task and that it is not only allowed but even recommended and eminently sensible to accept support from community members, voluntary and professional services. For moral reasons or out of a feeling of guilt or having high expectations of themselves, it seems to be hard for caring relatives to realize that it should be the responsibility of the local caring community to provide key information and give family carers the confidence to ask for further support (Harrop et al., 2014: 9).

Reflecting on 'care and gender justice': a 'hot potato'

Care work and the opportunities to receive care are unequally distributed in our societies, and this is also, or especially, the case in end-of-life care. In all focus groups with caring relatives (all females), either the overall care situation was characterized by this injustice, or micro-narratives have suggested an inequitable distribution of care or role conflicts among their family members. However, a too critical reflection of traditional gender roles, self-understandings, formative local cultures and public expectations threatens their identity and living concepts. Therefore the challenge is to trigger critical reflection in which one's own identity is not compromised. We consider reflecting care and gender inequity to be especially important because the care models supported by civil society – such as compassionate and caring communities – otherwise run the risk of reproducing social and gender-related inequity. Conversely, reflecting on these issues promotes the democratization of care.

Developing an 'organizational culture of dying'

One key challenge for improving end-of-life care is to establish a dignified culture of dying within organizations. There is much that can be done to change organizations and their cultures and structures towards the integration of a palliative care philosophy (Heimerl and Wegleitner, 2013). Thus organizational development in health care is an important precondition for community-based and needs-oriented end-of-life care. Although representatives of all social and healthcare organizations are participating in the project in Landeck, there is no specific focus on reorienting services and organizational culture. This could potentially form an obstacle to sustainability.

The absence of specialized palliative care as both an opportunity and a barrier

As indicated above, a conscious strategic decision was taken to implement the model project in a region where no specialized palliative care services are currently available (except coordinated hospice volunteers). It has been shown that in this way the responsibilities for end-of-life care are distributed broadly in the community, maybe because no clearly identified organization of 'dying experts' to which this could be delegated exists. However, with a view to project sustainability concerns, the absence of an established palliative care organization, required to anchor the subject, could also be a problem.

Hopes for the future

Governance for and of caring communities

One hope we associate with the project is to represent a model of good practice for community-oriented end-of-life care in German-speaking Europe. We furthermore hope to have an impact on prospective hospice and palliative care developments towards strengthening social space and community-oriented care practice and policy, that is 'public care' for frail, critically ill and dying people and their loved ones. The prerequisite for this would be that healthcare policy must establish new forms of governance (Conway, 2011), or governmentality (Foucault, 1991), to afford regional sustainable self-development in building compassionate communities. To this end, councils and regional authorities have to open up public spaces, and provide settings in which the persons concerned, civil society representatives and informal and formal caregivers have the opportunity to exchange existential experiences and knowledge, where the social ethical discourses about 'a good life', about care, solidarity, harm reduction, prevention and the common handling of vulnerability, life-limiting illness, dementia, frailty, dying, death and bereavement are encouraged. This is not a matter of one-sided political planning of palliative care services, but a cooperative, communal shaping of living and dying spaces in human solidarity, which must be placed in the forefront of governance.

From 'our' project to the caring communities culture and policy

It is currently not possible to predict how quickly and sustainably the community development process might shift from 'our common project' to a widely supported caring culture in Landeck and to a central initiative of its local policy. There is hope in the fact that various local actors and groups are increasingly taking on responsibility for launching initiatives and projects, and in the contribution of local officials with social affairs remits. Thus, for the immediate future we hope that this broad culture of engagement in the community of Landeck will continue, that the various initiatives will be implemented and that citizens will be involved to an even greater extent in gaining 'ownership' of and control over the caring community as an ongoing cultural process offering solidarity and compassion in living and dying.

> If there is to be a community in the world of individuals, it can only be (and it needs to be) a community woven together from sharing and mutual care; a community of concern and responsibility for the equal right to be human and the equal ability to act on that right.
> (Bauman, 2001: 149f.)

References

Abel, J., Walter, T., Carey, L.B. et al. (2013) Circles of care: should community development redefine the practice of palliative care? *BMJ Supportive & Palliative Care.* doi: 10.1136/bmjspcare-2012-000359.

Barry, V. and Patel, M. (2013) *An Overview of Compassionate Communities in England.* London: Murray Hall Community Trust; National Council for Palliative Care Dying Matters.

Bauman, Z. (2000) *Liquid Modernity.* Cambridge: Polity Press.

Bauman, Z. (2001) *Community. Seeking Safety in an Insecure World.* Cambridge: Polity Press.

Brundtland, G.H. (1989) Global change and our common future. *Environment* 31(5): 16–43.

Centeno, C., Lynch, T., Donea, O., Rocafort, J. and Clark, D. (2013) *EAPC Atlas of Palliative Care in Europe 2013.* Milan: EAPC Press.

Conway, S. (ed.) (2011) *Governing Death and Loss. Empowerment, Involvement, and Participation.* New York: Oxford University Press.

Council of Europe – European Health Committee (2003) *Recommendation Rec (2003) of the Committee of Ministers to member states on the organisation of palliative care.* Adopted by the Committee of Ministers on 12 November 2003 at the 860th meeting of the Ministers' Deputies.

Dooris, M. (1999) Healthy cities and Local Agenda 21: the UK experience – challenges for the new millennium. *Health Promotion International* 14(4): 365–375.

Dörner, K. (2007) *Leben und Sterben, wo ich hingehöre. Dritter Sozialraum und neues Hilfesystem.* Neumünster: Paranus Verlag.

European Association for Palliative Care (EAPC) (2009) White Paper on standards and norms for hospice and palliative care in Europe: part 1. Recommendations from the European Association for Palliative Care. *European Journal of Palliative Care* 09/16(6): 278–289.

Foucault, M. (1991) Governmentality. In: G. Burchell, C. Gordon and P. Miller (eds) *The Foucault Effect: Studies in Governmentality.* Hemel Hempstead: Harvester Wheatsheaf, 87–104.

Hancock, T. (1997) Healthy cities and communities: past, present, and future. *National Civic Review* 86(1): 11–21.

Hancock, T. (2001) People, partnerships and human progress: building community capital. *Health Promotion International* 16(3): 275–280.

Harrop, E., Byrne, A. and Nelson, A. (2014) 'It's alright to ask for help': findings from a qualitative study exploring the information and support needs of family carers at the end of life. *BMC Palliative Care* 13: 22, www.biomedcentral.com/1472-684X/13/22.

Heimerl, K. and Wegleitner, K. (2013) Organizational and health system change through participatory research. In: J. Hockley, K. Froggatt and K. Heimerl (eds) *Participatory Research in Palliative Care: Actions and Reflections.* Oxford: Oxford University Press, 27–39.

Heller, A. (1996) Sterben in Organisationen. In: R. Grossmann (ed.) *Gesundheitsförderung und Public Health. Öffentliche Gesundheit durch Organisation entwickeln.* Wien: Facultas, 214–231.

Hockley, J., Froggatt, K. and Heimerl, K. (eds) (2013) *Participatory Research in Palliative Care: Actions and Reflections*. Oxford: Oxford University Press.

Kellehear, A. (1999) *Health Promoting Palliative Care*. Melbourne: Oxford University Press.

Kellehear, A. (2005) *Compassionate Cities: Public Health and End-of-Life Care*. London: Routledge.

Kellehear, A. (2013) Compassionate communities: end-of-life care as everyone's responsibility. *QJM: An International Journal of Medicine*. doi: 10.1093/qjmed/hct200.

Kumar, S. (2007) Kerala, India: a regional community-based palliative care model. *Journal of Pain and Symptom Management* 33: 623–627.

Maddocks, I. (2003) The caring community. *Progress in Palliative Care* 11(4): 181–182. doi: http://dx.doi.org/10.1179/096992603225002618

Minkler, M. and Wallerstein, N. (eds) (2003) *Community-Based Participatory Research for Health*. San Francisco, CA: Jossey-Bass.

Nemeth, C. and Rottenhofer, I. (2004) *Abgestufte Hospiz- und Palliativversorgung in Österreich*. Wien: Österreichisches Bundesinstitut für Gesundheitswesen.

Nussbaum, M.C. (2003) *Upheavals of Thought: The Intelligence of Emotions*. Cambridge: Cambridge University Press.

Pelttari, L., Pissarek, H. and Zottele, P. (2014) *Hospiz und Palliative Care in Österreich*. Datenerhebung 2013. Dachverband Hospiz Österreich.

Rosenberg, J.P. and Yates, P.M. (2010) Health promotion in palliative care: the case for conceptual congruence. *Critical Public Health* 20(2): 201–210.

Rumbold, B. (2012) Public health approaches to palliative care in Australia. In: L. Sallnow, S. Kumar and A. Kellehear (eds) *International Perspectives on Public Health and Palliative Care*. London: Routledge, 52–68.

Sallnow, L. and Paul, S. (2014) Understanding community engagement in end-of-life care: developing conceptual clarity. *Critical Public Health*, doi: 10.1080/09581596.2014.909582

Sallnow, L., Kumar, S. and Kellehear, A. (eds) (2012) *International Perspectives on Public Health and Palliative Care*. London: Routledge.

Saunders, C. (2000) The evolution of palliative care. *Patient Education and Counseling* 41: 7–13.

Tronto, J.C. (2013) *Caring Democracy. Markets, Equality, and Justice*. New York: New York University Press.

Walter, T. (1999) A death in our street. *Health & Place* 5: 119–124.

WCED (World Commission on Environment and Development) (1987) *Our Common Future*. Oxford: Oxford University Press.

WHO – World Health Organization UNICEF (1978) *Primary Health Care: Report of the International Conference on Primary Health Care*. Alma-Ata, USSR, 6–12 September. Geneva: WHO.

WHO – World Health Organization (1986) Ottawa Charter for Health Promotion. *Health Promotion* 1(4): i–v.

WHO – World Health Organization (1990) *Cancer Pain Relief and Palliative Care. Report of a WHO Expert Committee*. Geneva: WHO.

9 'Ethics from the bottom up'

Promoting networks and participation through shared stories of care

Patrick Schuchter and Andreas Heller

In the region of Bad Bentheim (Lower Saxony, Germany), our project brings together the relatives of old and dying people, professionals from healthcare organizations and people from other living and working contexts in order to share their sorrows and care experiences. The aim is to create supportive environments and networks.

The political philosopher and care ethicist Joan Tronto (2013) suggests that a caring society and a caring democracy require settings where people can learn from and about the lives of others. The 'basic action' of a compassionate community is thus to create settings where people effectively have the opportunity to develop concerns and compassion for each other, to learn how to trace paths to a good life with and for others in the midst of suffering, and to identify gaps in the local care network. Volunteers are trained in workshops to become facilitators of existential dialogues and hold a key role in spreading the insights in the community, in and between healthcare and other relevant organizations. Thus, a collective learning process regarding care at the end of life and related existential issues is initiated through a participatory action research design. By this means, a new way of practising ethics in health care is realized – based on a care ethics and narrative approach that is quite different from the well-established paradigm of clinical ethics consultation. In opposition to the 'expert-driven dilemma-case-deliberation', this project is a realization of a very different approach – the exchange of meaningful care stories as an example of what we argue is the development of an 'ethics from the bottom up'. By promoting a compassionate community through shared narratives of care and concern, a paradigmatic shift from clinical ethics to 'communal' ethics is put into action.

In such a way, the fundamentals and sources of the philosophy of the project, which we will discuss closer in the following, are manifold. On the one hand, they are rooted in a deeper understanding of hospice and palliative care, while, on the other hand, developments around the compassionate community strategy are taken up. From our perspective, both concepts and movements are grounded in a fundamental ethics of care, which provides new impulses for a 'caring democracy' (Tronto, 2013) or the 'democratisation of care' but at the same time requires a new form of ethical deliberation. We are on the way to a 'care revolution'.

Hospice and palliative care

Palliative care originates from the international hospice movement, whose implementation in German-speaking countries began with a slight delay – arriving behind their English and American counterparts in the 1980s. Within the framework of international euthanasia societies (the right-to-die movement, DGHS = Deutsche Gesellschaft für Humanes Sterben) calling for dignified death, for the purposes of criminal law and legalizing active euthanasia, and in the context of rapid development of highly specialized and technology-dominated medicine, it seemed impossible to have a dignified death in a hospital: The image of a 'cold lonely death in a broom closet' was overwhelming. This provided a focus for the hospice movement, with the objective of being able to die in dignity and character, among the people concerned and affected.

The hospice concept continues to live on under the idea of European and ancient oriental hospitality. Human life, conceived as a pilgrimage, is reliant on hospitality to find its path and destination. Hospices offer hospitality without an ulterior motive – they provide unconditional interest in others and for the sake of others in their own right. Such hospices are not just buildings, but rather represent an approach and attitude to people and culture in society. In times of increasing commercialization and managerialism of health care ('It only counts if you can count it!'), the hospice currently provides a critically different option in offering care and attention to people in need via assistance and support for end-of-life requirements. First and foremost, the hospice movement is simply a citizens' movement, supported by volunteers – dedicated people committed to the right and the opportunity for all to have a good, dignified and individualized death at the end of life, regardless of religion, race, gender and financial status. In the German-speaking countries, palliative care (in Germany translated as *palliative medicine*) had eventually become marked by a profound process of professionalization, dominated by medicalization and institutionalization, an approach that is still very influential today.

According to the globally accepted definition of the World Health Organization (WHO), palliative care is,

> an approach by which the quality of life of patients and their families will be improved if they are faced with a life-threatening illness and its associated problems. This shall be achieved through the prevention and relief of suffering by means of early identification, faultless assessment and treatment of pain and other physical, psychosocial and spiritual problems.

> (WHO, 2002)

This definition includes the focused involvement of relatives and carers – that is, of persons affected by the suffering and of those connected to them – and sharing in their concerns and care. Particular attention is given to the grief, which sets in not only after death, but often also over the lengthy period of the diagnosis of a chronic disease, the multiple treatments until death, and the time beyond.

In the revised version of the original definition, dating back to 1990, it is clearly emphasized that the palliative care approach should be applied very early on within the disease process – indeed, in parallel with other curative measures (WHO, 2002). It remains open as to how these conceptual building blocks are to be implemented within different healthcare systems: thus, a variety of structures and forms have developed in Germany, Austria and Switzerland over the past 20 years.

A starting point is to look at the linkage and interweaving of the development of individuals with the development of organizations; this is based on the view that a culture respecting death is always an *organizational* culture respecting death (Heller, 2000). Hospice work and palliative care, especially in German-speaking countries, are viewed as healthcare concepts focused on different emphases.

In the development of the hospice concept, the applicability of these conceptual elements for the chronically ill and elderly was never strictly excluded – indeed they were even decidedly highlighted by Cicely Saunders: 'Terminal care should not be a facet of oncology, but of geriatric medicine, neurology, general practice and throughout medicine' (Saunders and Baines, 1983: 2).

Nevertheless, the concept was based on and developed for terminally-ill individuals with cancer. Academic palliative medicine has been largely rooted within the context of university oncology. There are, however, many other groups of affected persons (only about 25 per cent of people in Central Europe die from a tumour-based disease, with 75 per cent dying from something else altogether). The focus of attention in the last few years has been, in particular, on the deaths of older men and women. There have been pilot projects trying to establish a hospice and palliative culture in nursing homes (Heller and Kittelberger, 2010), and for several years now there has been a systematic dedication in palliative care discourse at the international level, focusing on other target groups, including older persons.

Creating a close link between gerontology and palliative care, Seymour and Hanson (2001: 102) write:

> Both attend to the pursuit of symptom control, while advising the judicious use of investigations and rejecting highly invasive and aggressive treatment modalities; both make the person and their family the unit of care, and have led the way in developing multidisciplinary and community-based models of care. In so doing they have developed parallel discourses of 'patient-centred' care, 'quality of life', 'dignity'

and 'autonomy'. Further, both disciplines focus on areas – ageing and cancer – that tend to provoke strong, even 'phobic' reactions from the public at large.

A WHO publication entitled 'Better Palliative Care for Older People' (Davies and Higginson, 2004) is showing the way. This calls for public health strategies at the national level, with the objective of improving palliative care for older people. The term *palliative geriatrics* has been experimented with in German-speaking countries, and it certainly implies a 'medicalising tendency' (Clark, 2002). It does not accommodate appropriately either the practice or the daily lives of the elderly, or the interdisciplinary theoretical reflection of the concerns and care of the elderly.

The revolutionary notion in this approach of a new end-of-life care culture views the individual person, as a woman, man, child or adolescent (see children's hospice movement; Knapp and Madden, 2012), within the context of their life relationships. The 'care unit' is therefore the social system, not just the individual.

According to the concepts and 'discovery' of Cicely Saunders, people suffer *comprehensively* (her concept of 'total pain') – that is, bio-psycho-socially and spiritually. This multidimensionality in the anthropology of 'caring' is indeed a revolution, which is not only represented by conventional medicine. It renders interdisciplinary theory and practice essential, as a logical consequence designed to complement inter-professionalism, especially for the so-called voluntary workers, the citizens (in a civic concept of civil society) who maintain the continuity of care.

Palliative care can be understood as an innovation within the healthcare system, and as both an organizational and a social innovation: interdisciplinary theory and practice are essential in the palliative care concept, while the 'unit of care' is not just the individual, but the social system as a whole. The multidimensionality in the anthropology of 'caring' (on bio-psycho-social and spiritual levels) can be seen as a revolutionary notion in this new care culture, where so-called voluntary workers and 'civil society' maintain the continuity of care.

The hospice and palliative care concept is also relevant for the knowledge society, because knowledge is not created by the experts or professionals, but by the laypeople. It is an anti-elitist approach, in which professionals act as supporters and facilitators, focusing on the needs of the persons concerned.

Insofar as hospice work and palliative care have been creating a profound innovation within the healthcare system – and because this gap has been discovered and revealed as the 'place for action' – the movement, as such, is guided by interdisciplinary, inter-professional, inter-organizational, interreligious and intercultural principles (Heller, 2007).

Interestingly, hospice work is also an area in which a new image of a 'healthy death' (Wenzel, 2012) can be created. Death is understood and attended to not as a result of disease or organ failure, but as part of the (spiritual) developmental process of a person, wherein pain may also be considered as an approach to a central dimension of life. 'Healing' may then be possible, even if 'curing' no longer is (Rakel and Weil, 2003).

In this sense, hospice work and palliative care serve as a thorn in the side of the medically- and curatively-oriented healthcare system, demanding a challenging discussion about death despite all the achievements of modern medicine not only for the dying individual but equally for the relatives, carers and professionals involved. Hospice work and palliative care not only remind us but can also bring us (as a society) back to the power of civil society, which is concerned to form and participate in new 'cultures of care'.

The importance of ethical deliberation in promoting compassionate communities

It is a historical merit and a substantial contribution of public health and of health promotion approaches to have put questions of health and illness, as well as of dying, loss and grief, in a wider and more fundamental perspective. Both with regard to curative medicine and with regard to professional-oriented palliative care, it is claimed that health or the alleviation and prevention of suffering in dying and grieving are not created for instance in hospitals or nursing homes but more fundamentally 'where people learn, work, play, and love', as it was articulated in the Ottawa Charter (WHO, 1986); and also, we need to add, where people grow old, mourn and have to cope with the finitude of life. In the end, the pursuit of health and the attempts to ease suffering caused by losses lead to the question of which collective form we want to give to our life and our life conditions.

Therefore, two important insights should be noted. First, the change in perspective towards public health points of view not only broadens the scientific and disciplinary basis (for instance from medicine to psychology, sociology, etc.) but, more significantly, means that the logic of dealing with substantial social questions through scientific expertise is transcended. If questions of health and dying are widened and deepened to such an extent that they can no longer be distinguished from the ethical question of 'the good life', then the 'limits of science' (Buchanan, 2000: 49–70) are reached. This widening and deepening of the question of health has found a masterful expression in Aaron Antonovsky's central metaphor of the *good swimmer*: 'The twin question is: How dangerous is our river? How well can we swim?' (Antonovsky, 1996, 14). Since Socrates and Hellenistic philosophy, philosophers have posed the ethical question through an analogy between a specialist art (e.g. swimming) and the art of living in general (Sellars, 2009). Moreover, in the same tradition there is no doubt that the art of living cannot be separated from the art of dying, as famously expressed in a few sentences from Seneca: 'Throughout the whole of life, one must continue to learn to live and what will amaze you even more, throughout life you must learn to die' (Seneca, *On the Shortness of Life*). And, we may add, we must learn how to create social life, and environmental conditions.

The necessity of 'an ethic for health promotion' has been strongly and very clearly expressed by David Buchanan. The crucial point of his argument, it seems to us, should consequently be taken seriously in compassionate community strategies or civil society-oriented hospice work. The argument goes as follows: in the field of public health and health promotion,

> the kinds of health problems now facing the field have shifted, but our thinking about how to respond to them has not shifted accordingly. The leading health problems of the day have shifted from infectious diseases to chronic 'lifestyle' diseases. The locus of responsibility has thus shifted from invasive microorganisms to human volitions, but the framework for thinking about how to deal with these problems has not changed. It is still a paradigm of power, mastery, and control.
>
> (Buchanan, 2000: 4)

Health promotion interventions seek to change attitudes, behaviour and circumstances – and the success of interventions is measured or evaluated by various indicators of (a change of) health status. If, however, the 'objects' of interventions are questions of lifestyle (choices) and the shaping of the life-world, then not only scientific methods are 'incapable of providing answers to normative questions' (Buchanan, 2000: 4), for instance 'whether it is worth sacrificing one's (physical) health for a social cause' (Buchanan, 2000: 61). On the contrary, it is morally dubious to influence attitudes, behaviour and circumstances by methods whose strength is to predict and to control. At worst, a simple orientation via a health status indicator model and effective behaviour change methods 'undermines the most fundamental understanding of ethical human relationship' (Buchanan 2000: 4).

In other words, the 'first' intervention in health promotion or health promoting palliative care programmes is to organize an open process of discussion and deliberation for and with citizens which offers the possibility and a public space in which to think about what counts in life, and about sorrows and concerns that people have and feel. The first step to promote health, for civil society-oriented hospice work or for promoting compassionate communities is to organize ethical deliberations in this sense – the common and most profound ethical goal of these social movements is to promote the self-enlightenment of individuals and the social systems they are living in, oriented at a good life (until the last) with and for others in just institutions (Ricoeur, 1990: 199).

The importance of compassionate communities for the further development of ethical deliberation: from clinical ethics to communal 'ethics from the bottom up'

If, on the one hand, it has to be said that promoting health or compassionate communities starts with a process of ethical reflection of citizens, it must equally be said, on the other hand, that current methods and concepts of applied and organized ethical deliberation (or ethics 'consultation') are not qualified and able to fulfil the requirements of ethical questions in the field of health promotion and health promoting palliative care. The predominant model of ethical deliberation in healthcare settings, the clinical ethics consultation, is designed for the specific orientation needs of curative medicine. The analogous step from medicine to health promotion, from professionalist palliative care to compassionate communities has not been carried out in ethics. It is worth taking a closer look, for a start, at such paradigmatic displacements in ethics at a more conceptual level.

The standard model of ethical deliberation: clinical ethics consultation

Today, we can talk of a *standard model* of ethics in healthcare organizations. Central to the standard model is the establishment of a healthcare ethics committee within an organization. The main function of the ethics committee, besides the education of staff and development of policies and guidelines, is to offer clinical ethics consultation. This means providing 'clinicians with an analytic framework for identifying and resolving ethical dilemmas that arise in the clinical setting' (Post et al., 2007: 137). According to this understanding, ethics comes into play when a moral dilemma occurs during medical treatment processes, for example in the context of end-of-life care or in the context of refusal of treatment. Ethical issues are moral dilemmas in decision making – in the context of curative or palliative medicine. Let us say furthermore – which is well supported by the literature – that within the standard model of ethical deliberation, a pivotal role is normally ascribed to the four principles of bioethics as identified by Beauchamp and Childress (autonomy, non-maleficence, beneficence, justice). It is indeed the definition of a moral dilemma when core ethical principles and consequently the obligations of clinicians are in conflict. Normally, the reference to these ethical principles directs and structures the perception of an ethical problem. The principles serve to guide the course of the deliberation and finally to justify decisions and measures taken after having balanced the different obligations. Finally, in the standard model, a deliberation or consultation setting is set up when a dilemma, an ethical emergency, has occurred – which is at least true for *prospective* case deliberation – and it is organized as a particular and independent form of communication different from other forms of communication.

These are the main characteristics of ethics consultation within the framework of the clinical standard model: moral dilemmas as subject of deliberation, orientation along normative principles, treatment decisions as the objective of ethics consultation, and organization of the deliberation as a special communication in case of ethical emergency. Without denying the utility and the merits of the standard model, it can be argued, however, that conceiving ethics in this way also means reducing ethics. The focus on normative principles, decisions and dilemma-situations as isolated events obscures many possible deliberation processes, which should also be perceived as ethical issues and ethical deliberations.

The art of living and dying

The British-born, Ghanaian/American philosopher Kwame Anthony Appiah, for example, criticizes the focus on moral dilemmas and refers to this narrowing tendency in modern ethics as a 'dilemma-dilemma' (Appiah, 2009: 198). He points out that according to a long philosophical tradition, key ethical issues deal with everyday life and with life as a whole from a reflective and evaluative perspective. Ethical issues concern questions such as success or failure of our life plans, the possibility of self-respect and of participation in institutions of a community. They also deal with the meaningfulness or meaninglessness of our actions and experiences, and with issues like love, friendship and how to deal with passions. With special regard to palliative care, we could say: ethics is about living with one's own vulnerability, with the fear of death, pain and suffering, and living with experiences of loss. Basically, ethics is about the art of living and dying.

From this point of view, the ethics of dilemma circles too closely around the isolated question of what to *do* in this particular case of ethical emergency – comparable to an express repair service. The essential ethical questions are not so much solutions of dilemma situations as the *fundamental questions of human existence,* which come to the fore particularly in borderline situations of weakness, dependency and illness, and when facing death. Ethics is not just about single actions, but also about the lives of the actors. Philosophical reflection does not so much serve as a normative evaluation, but can be seen as an 'exercise' (Sellars, 2009).

Ethics of care

Being in a situation of suffering (normally) implies falling into a deep existential crisis regarding fundamental life questions. Not only does a biological dysfunction require medical cure or the relief of physical pain, and a 'self-care deficit' not only requires nursing. Above all, the wounded existence requires *care* – care in order to repair the relationship with oneself, with others and with the world; to reconcile oneself with failure, negativity and death. The situation of suffering requires a relationship with oneself and the world, in which death, pain, vulnerability, dependency and grief occupy a thus far unknown and now intrusive role in one's own life. In such a situation, the most basic question of ethics is not so much about the non-violation of norms (or the breach of professional obligations), but about the question as it has been articulated by the Danish philosopher and medical doctor Peter Kemp (1987: 69): Is there some kind of happiness possible in the midst of suffering or in spite of suffering? Is it possible to gain some kind of happiness for the suffering or the dying? The medical sociologist Arthur Frank reminds us that even 'the traditional ideal of medicine is to offer more than treatment': 'before and after fundamental medicine offers diagnoses, drugs, and surgery to those who suffer, it should offer consolation' (Frank, 2004: 2). This is probably the best definition of happiness in the midst of suffering: consolation. By consolation we cannot get rid of the causes of pain and suffering but we can – so to speak – overcome the suffering from suffering, elevate the soul and its reactions above illness and pain, at least for one precious moment. Perhaps this is also the contribution of compassionate communities and of hospice work for society as a whole: the search for consolation against isolation, offering the vision of a non-trivial happiness.

The logic of *care* is quite different from the way of thinking in mainstream ethics and subsequently in mainstream ethics consultation, including the (implicit) basic anthropological assumptions. In contrast to prevailing modern ethical theory, as it has been shaped by philosophers like Kant, Rawls or by discourse theory, care ethics do not focus on autonomous, rational individuals who subsequently cooperate in the form of contract-relations. The modern view on what constitutes human beings – and thus the modern way of constructing society and the public sphere – can be described as an 'ontological individualism'. Care ethics remind us that through many phases of life we are anything other than reasonable, autonomous or independent individuals: in childhood, old age, sickness and weakness. On the contrary, from a care ethics perspective, it is indispensable to understand ourselves as fundamentally connected beings. The basic action of human growth (growth of persons, communities and the society as a whole) consists of 'caring'.

It should be noted that in principle, relationships of care are asymmetric – nevertheless they are mutual. Care relationships are both: helpful to the care-receiver and at least potentially 'existentially' rewarding for the caregiver. To care for others means personal growth – not least through obtaining (rather 'tacit') knowledge and insights on the finiteness of human condition, on life and death in a proper 'philosophical' sense (cf. Ricoeur, 1990: 313).

Learning from others through stories of care and concern

Thus, ethics comprises two efforts or 'arts', which are closely related with each other and which are both derived from the two lines mentioned above: ethics as the art of living and the ethics of care: the effort and the art of *understanding* a person in his or her reality of suffering, which means entering with others into *compassionate and caring relations*; and the effort or the art of searching for and perhaps discovering *possibilities of a good life (or consolation in dying and in mourning) in suffering with and for others.* From this point of view, treatment decisions are only *one* part – namely the case of ethical emergency – of a continuing process of reflection and dialogue. This process challenges the practical wisdom of both the suffering and the carer. Ethics is a learning process. From Socrates to contemporary philosophers like Paul Ricoeur, the tradition of ethics keeps reminding us that ethical learning is not a business of lonely (autonomous) individuals but a matter of giving and receiving between related persons – even if a situation initially appears to be asymmetric. *If* persons are willing to enter into an ethical learning process, then the stories of suffering persons may help them to reflect upon their own life experiences. And vice versa, suffering persons may benefit from a reflected life experience that enables others to understand them in a non-superficial manner. As has been said in the context of a narrative approach to ethics: stories of borderline situations at their best represent models of consolation and the possibility of traces of happiness despite misfortune. These stories are 'the first laboratory of moral judgement' (Ricoeur, 1990: 167).

Paradigmatic shifts

In summary, a change from expert-driven clinical ethics to communal ethics from the bottom up implies the following displacements: First, subjects of ethical deliberations are not just dilemma situations but meaningful experiences and situations in general, which concern the fundamental questions of human life. Second, the 'basic action' of ethical deliberation is not a principle-based reflection on a 'case' represented primarily in medical facts but it rather involves thinking about everyday existential issues on the basis of paradigmatic stories and connecting with other people by making an effort to understand and to feel with others. By giving narratives (stories) the status of the central language-game in ethical deliberation, the dominance of expert knowledge is annulled in favour of a democratization of the opportunities to speak and a consequent participation (for instance, by relatives). Third, the essential question is less how to balance obligations or norms but how to trace paths to a good life in the midst of suffering with and for others. Furthermore, the objective of ethical deliberation is not just a singular decision but the sustainable cultivation of collective practical wisdom in a web of meaningful relationships. And, finally, ethics will be organized on everyday ethical reflection, situated in everyday practice in organizations, communities and so on – and not just when a moral dilemma occurs.

'Ethics from the bottom up' – experiences from a project in Lower Saxony (Germany)

The central idea of the project is to organize and to translate into concrete processes ethical 'deliberation', by which people can learn from and about the lives of others through narratives, share their sorrows and concerns, connect or mutually come into contact beyond social roles, different life-worlds or organizational borders, and try to find ways to lead a good life in the midst of suffering. The aim is to establish roundtables – according to the possibilities and requirements of the respective setting and context – so that people can bring their sorrows and concerns to the table, share and discuss these and develop perspectives on how to deal with certain challenges.

A first and exemplary realization of communal 'ethics from the bottom up' is taking place in the rural district of Grafschaft Bentheim, which is a small district in the south-west part of Lower Saxony (Germany), with approximately 133,400 inhabitants. With regard to palliative care, the region is characterized by a high supply density with nursing, elderly care and hospice services. There are 21 nursing homes, more than 20 care services for the elderly and one hospital in Nordhorn, the district seat of Bentheim. Project partner initiators in the region are a nursing home and the local hospice service. The hospice service (*Hospiz Hilfe Grafschaft Bentheim e.V.*) is one of the largest hospice services in Lower Saxony. It has existed for more than 10 years and has over 500 members, 90 of which are active volunteers, and three staff coordinators. The hospice service Grafschaft Bentheim accompanies about 150–200 persons per year. The nursing home of St. Vincenz (*St. Vincenz Haus GmbH*) has 52 nursing places and is maintained by the Catholic Parish of '*Mariä Himmelfahrt*' in Neuenhaus. A good and close working cooperation exists between the nursing home and the hospice service, as well as a cooperation agreement.

In the project sponsored by the Robert-Bosch Stiftung Stuttgart, a steering committee has been established and consists of the initiating institutions together with management personnel from different palliative and elderly care services and institutions. The balance between competition and cooperation is a challenge in certain respects, but, according to the metaphor of a 'common infection with the hospice virus', a shared interest and philosophy has been expressed. In concrete terms, this common will and understanding should be translated into an offer of support for family carers and relatives of severely ill, old and dying persons.

In the sense of promoting compassionate communities, it can be said that the project enables the reorientation of healthcare services that have so far offered individual–holistic palliative care (Kellehear and Young, 2011: 90f.)

towards networking and orientation along the perspectives, sorrows and concerns of citizens – which, in our context, means becoming familiar with the perspectives of family carers and relatives.

The heart of the project consists of several workshops where volunteers are trained in facilitating existential dialogues and undertaking the existential dialogues themselves in different settings and contexts. Participants of the workshops are in the first instance volunteers from the hospice service and members of staff from nursing homes and from different nursing services in the community. There is an astonishingly high level of interest in the project, and about 80 persons participated in the first workshop. This remarkable level of participation could be interpreted as a sign that a deficit of professional services, which only respond insufficiently to psycho-social and spiritual–philosophical implications of illness and frailty in working routines, is keenly felt.

In the workshop, we propose dialogue forms which are much less structured than strictly linear dialogue guides and a little more structured than some free impulse questions. The idea is to open the dialogue and thus to enable and to allow others to tell their story more easily. People approach each other and discover similarities and differences. Telling stories of care creates connectedness, relief and new perspectives. A first dialogue form (the emphasis in Workshop I) and a documentation form aim at generating, sharing and documenting care stories (about the concerns and sorrows of relatives and family carers), relating insights and feelings, as well as suggestions for improvements in the region, the organizations or the community. We use impulse questions such as the following:

1   Which story of care (a situation, an experience) remains in your memory and is for this reason important and touching?
2   What is astonishing about this story? Which feelings, inner images, thoughts and insights arise? What is the underlying theme of the story?
3   Which practical conclusions can be drawn from the stories and the insights in the dialogue?

A second dialogue form (the emphasis in Workshop II) comprises a suggestion of how to reflect upon and discuss in more depth certain recurring themes from the stories. Questions and orientation guide for the dialogue still remain simple and elementary:

1   What have been your experiences concerning this issue? Also think of other areas of life where these issues arise: which insights can be transferred? Do not focus on solutions and actions but try to deepen the descriptions.
2   Which practical conclusions can be drawn from the insights and experiences in the dialogue?

Special attention will be paid (the emphasis in Workshop III) to reflecting upon the dialogues and the documentation as a social process in the region. Here are the relevant questions:

1   Who should engage in an existential dialogue with whom? Which persons in which social roles and from which life-worlds?
2   Who – in his or her social role – should hear and listen to insights, concerns, stories and questions arising from the dialogues?

As the project is in progress at the time of writing, the first workshop has taken place so far, as well as the first existential dialogues in different contexts, organized and facilitated by the members in the workshop. Twelve dialogues were undertaken (excluding dialogues during the workshop), and participants were relatives or family carers of old, severely ill and other persons, who were in part old persons themselves, members of staff from the respective institutions and volunteers from the hospice service. Forty-five care short stories (excluding 20 stories from the workshop itself) are documented. Emerging themes concern questions of guilt, the burden of caring, lack of recognition for carers, living and making decisions under uncertainty, intense relationship dynamics, profound changes in personality, and others.

This represents the status of the project to the present date. With the next steps to be taken, the first results will be presented to the steering committee and to the participants in the second workshop. On this basis, the existential dialogues and the social process of networking coupled with the dialogues will be developed further in a participatory process.

Perpectives

We observe a new and simple way to bring relatives into communication with each other and with professional and (specialized) health services. This is one way of initiating the democratization of care, of finding support in the challenges of weakness and dying and building bridges to the medical doctors to invite them to take part in a partnership-driven communication. Already now questions concerning the sustainable establishment of the dialogues are discussed in the steering committee. The fact that in some facilities two or more existential dialogues have taken place during the first period of the project may be interpreted as a positive sign. There are some difficulties for mobile care services in the organization of group meetings, so that person-to-person dialogues have been organized instead. The project has an explorative character, and thus is open to a variety of organizational forms of the dialogues. In any case, it is already apparent at this time that theoretical and practical fundamentals for a communal ethics from the bottom up have been outlined – and thus for a new form of ethical deliberation which is qualified to meet the requirements of ethical questions in the field of health promoting palliative care and of promoting compassionate communities.

References

Antonovsky, A. (1996) The salutogenic model as a theory to guide health promotion. *Health Promotion International* 11(1): 11–18.

Appiah, A.K. (2009) *Ethische Experimente*. München: Beck.

Beauchamp, T.L. and Childress, J.F. (2001) *Principles of Biomedical Ethics*. New York: Oxford University Press.

Buchanan, D. (2000) *An Ethic for Health Promotion. Rethinking the Sources of Human Well-Being*. New York: Oxford University Press.

Clark, D. (2002) *Between hope and acceptance: the medicalisation of dying. BMJ* 324: 904–907.

Davies, E. and Higginson, I. (2004) *Better Palliative Care for Older People*. WHO Regional Office for Europe. WHO.

Frank, A.W. (2004) *The Renewal of Generosity. Illness, Medicine, and How to Live*. Chicago, IL: Chicago University Press.

Heller, A. (2007) Die Einmaligkeit von Menschen verstehen und bis zuletzt bedienen. Palliative Versorgung und ihre Prinzipien. In: A. Heller, K. Heimerl and S. Husebø (eds) *Wenn nichts mehr zu machen ist, ist noch viel zu tun. Wie alte Menschen würdig sterben können*, pp. 191–220. Freiburg im Breisgau: Lambertus.

Heller, A. and Kittelberger, F. (2010) *Hospizkompetenz und Palliative Care im Alter. Eine Einführung*. Freiburg im Breisgau: Lambertus.

Heller, B. (2000) Kulturen des Sterbens. Interreligiosität als Herausforderung für Palliative Care. In: A. Heller, K. Heimerl and C. Metz (eds) *Kultur des Sterbens. Bedingungen für das Lebensende gestalten*, pp. 177–192. Freiburg im Breisgau: Lambertus.

Kellehear, A. and Young, B. (2011) Resilient communities. In: S. Conway (ed.) *Governing Death and Loss. Empowerment, Involvement, and Participation*, pp. 89–98. New York: Oxford University Press.

Kemp, P. (1987) *Ethique et Médicine*. Paris: Tierce.

Knapp, C. and Madden, V. (eds) (2012) *Pediatric Palliative Care: Global Perspectives*. Dordrecht: Springer.

Post, L.F., Blustein, J. and Dubler, N.N. (2007) *Handbook for Health Care Ethics Committees*. Baltimore, MD: Johns Hopkins University Press.

Rakel, D. and Weil, A. (2003) Philosophy of integrative medicine. In: D. Rakel (ed.) *Integrative Medicine*, pp. 3–10. Philadelphia, PA: Saunders.

Rawls, J. (1971) *A theory of justice*. Boston, Mass.: Belknap Press.

Ricoeur, P. (1990) *Soi-même comme un autre*. Paris: Seuil.

Saunders, C. and Baines, M. (1983) *Living with Dying: The Management of Terminal Disease*. Oxford: Oxford University Press.

Sellars, J. (2009) *The Art of Living. The Stoics on the Art and Function of Philosophy*, 2nd edn. London: Duckworth/Bristol Classical Paperbacks.

Seneca, L.A. (n.d.) *On the Shortness of Life*. Translated by John W. Basore. Loeb Classical Library. London: William Heinemann, 1932. Corpus scriptorum latinorum, a digital library of Latin literature: www.forumromanum.org/literature/seneca_younger/brev_e.html (Accessed 14 October 2014).

Seymour, J.E. and Hanson, E. (2001) Palliative care and older people. In: M. Nolan, S. Davies and G. Grant (eds) *Working with Older People and their Families*, pp. 99–119. Maidenhead: Open University Press.

Tronto, J. (2013) *Caring Democracy. Markets, Equality, and Justice*. New York: New York University Press.

Wenzel, C. (2012) Heil Sterben. Alternative Ansätze für eine ganzheitliche Begleitung Sterbender in Hospizarbeit und Palliative Care – *Band VI Schriftenreihe des Wissenschaftlichen Beirats im DHPV e.V.* Ludwigsburg: der hospiz Verlag.

World Health Organization (WHO) (1986) *Ottawa Charter for Health Promotion*. Geneva: WHO.

World Health Organization (WHO) (2002) *National Cancer Control Programmes. Policies and Managerial Guidelines*. Geneva: WHO.

10 Dementia-friendly pharmacy

A doorway in the community in Vienna and Lower Austria

Petra Plunger, Verena Tatzer, Katharina Heimerl and Elisabeth Reitinger

Compassionate communities and community pharmacies

It might come as a surprise to read about community pharmacies in this book dedicated to issues related to death and dying in 'compassionate communities'. Clearly, the focus here is on communities, their resources and organizational structures, and their procedures aiming at 'increas(ing) their community's resilience, support, and openness toward those affected by death, dying, and loss' (Barry and Patel, 2013).

Inspired by the Ottawa Charter for Health Promotion (World Health Organization and Welfare Canada, 1986), which is a major point of reference also for the 'Compassionate Communities' (Kellehear, 2005), we would like to propose that communities – if we talk about regionally defined settings – consolidate various settings such as schools, workplaces and healthcare organizations like community pharmacies, all of which might be included in a compassionate communities approach.

It is from this starting point that in this chapter the issue of dementia-friendly community pharmacies will be described, as a frame of reference. To outline some starting points of the project, a brief overview will be given on the situation of (community-based) dementia care in German-speaking countries, as well as on the health and social care system in Austria and its uptake of issues related to dementia. Next, the project 'Dementia-friendly Community Pharmacy' will be introduced – its methodology and interim results, and some lessons learned so far. We conclude by discussing some implications for further engagement of healthcare settings like community pharmacies in the development of compassionate communities.

Community care for people living with dementia and their caregivers in German-speaking countries

The situation in Austria: fragmentation of health and social care

It is estimated that there are around 100,000 individuals with dementia living in Austria today (Austrian Alzheimer Society, 2010). If we take into consideration that there are at least three to four family members immediately involved in the care, we can conclude that the issue concerns between 300,000 and 400,000 people in Austria, representing approximately 5 per cent of the population.

There is an extended and controversial debate in Austria and in the entire German-speaking world as to whether the care for people with dementia is primarily a professional task (e.g. Austrian Alzheimer Society, 2010; Kojer and Schmidl, 2011) or whether it concerns civil society and the community (Gröning and Heimerl, 2012; Wißmann and Gronemeyer, 2008).

The Austrian dementia strategy is on its way

Political attention for the important issue of care for persons with dementia has been paid in Austria through the publication of different dementia reports and recommendations for action by the two ministries concerned: the 'Dementia Handbook' was issued by the Ministry of Social Affairs and Consumer Protection in 2008. The 'First Austrian Dementia Report' was edited by the Public Health Insurance in 2009. There is a regularly issued 'Consensus Statement' edited by the Austrian Alzheimer Society, which is the medical society in this field in Austria (Austrian Alzheimer Society, 2006, 2010). The Austrian Federal Ministry of Health has published two brochures with recommendations for action (BMG, 2011, 2013) that pay particular attention to gender aspects.

Many European countries have elaborated dementia strategies (for an overview see www.alzheimer-europe.org/Policy-in-Practice2/National-Dementia-Plans). To date, there is no dementia strategy in Austria, although the design of such a strategy is currently in progress. The task force consists of experts from both the healthcare and the social care systems. Nevertheless the first results show a clear emphasis on medical issues. The discussion around an Austrian dementia strategy is dominated by the view that the care for people with dementia and the support of their caregivers in Austria is primarily a multi-professional task. Among the professionals, the medical perspective prevails. At the present time there is a considerable risk that the critique (Kellehear, 2009) that has been published concerning the NICE/SCIE (2006) Guidelines on Dementia in the UK will apply to the Austrian strategy as well.

Dementia-friendly community – a social movement?

There is also a second approach in Austria that postulates that the care for people with dementia and the support of their caregivers in Austria is primarily a community task. Inspired by the German discourse led by 'Aktion Demenz' (Dementia Action) (see Chapter 13 in this volume), there is the beginning of a movement in Austria that sees the care for people living with dementia primarily as an issue that concerns civil society.

There are a few model projects that adopt the civil society approach, such as 'Dementia-friendly third district in Vienna' and 'Dementia Action Vorarlberg'. Relatives and caregivers have founded a considerable number of self-help groups that are gathered within the umbrella organization 'Alzheimer Austria' (AA). AA sees itself as an advocate for those people affected and their relatives. Our project, 'Dementia-friendly Community Pharmacy', constitutes a relevant contribution to this approach in Austria.

Palliative care, health promotion and dementia

Dementia can be considered to be incurable, since it reduces life expectancy. Grief and bereavement are relevant issues for those affected. Palliative care plays an important role in dementia care (Small et al., 2008; Blasi et al., 2002). Many of these issues are discussed under the title 'Palliative Geriatrics' (Kojer and Schmidl, 2011) in Austria.

Likewise, health promotion offers some promising approaches when focusing on community-based dementia care: following the Ottawa Charter (1986), 'health promotion demands coordinated action by all concerned', be it individuals or groups, from different sectors of society. Therefore, in the course of the project, 're-orienting pharmacies' is one aim, as well as 'strengthening community action' and 'building individual skills'. We believe that participation of relevant actors and people concerned in all phases of the project is vitally important in order to reach these goals and form the basis for empowerment.

Developing dementia-friendly community pharmacies: guiding principles and main activities

In the following section, main aspects of the 'Dementia-friendly Community Pharmacy' project will be outlined, based on the considerations on community-based dementia care described above. First, a brief overview of community pharmacies in Austria – the legal and institutional framework and their tasks – will be given. Second, main principles in participatory health research, upon which the project is based, will be introduced. Following this line of argument, the experiences of caregivers and community pharmacy staff regarding dementia care in community pharmacies will be presented, as well as key interventions and project steps undertaken so far.

Organization and tasks of community pharmacies in Austria and potentials for dementia-friendly community work

In Austria the pharmacy system, as part of the health system, comes within the federal government's area of responsibilities, regulated by the Pharmacies Act, which sets out the legal underpinnings of pharmacies, and the Medicinal Products Act, which regulates the supply of medicines. The community pharmacy is a privately owned business with a public supply mandate: as of 2013, there were 1,344 community pharmacies operating in Austria. A community pharmacy reaches a broad spectrum of the population, with a disproportionately high share of older people and women. The main responsibility of a community pharmacy is to provide medicines to the general population, which includes the management of pharmacotherapy, health education and counselling (Austrian Chamber of Pharmacists, 2014).

Community pharmacies offer some possibilities for dementia care reaching the broad population and potentially also marginalized groups (Blenkinsopp, 2000): they are frequently the first contact with the health system, and the profession enjoys high levels of trust based on their expert status and competence. There is a high frequency of contacts with few barriers to access, as community pharmacies are located within the community with no appointments necessary, and a short waiting time. Contacts very often take place on a regular basis. Barriers include the 'medical gaze' of community pharmacists, as well as the business environment which might lead to loss of privacy and the intention to sell products conflicting with professional issues (Haslbeck and Schaeffer, 2009).

Health promotion and palliative care are not explicitly defined as part of the role of the community pharmacist in Austria. However, elements of these can be found in daily professional activities like giving advice, counselling on medications and self-medication, and health education.

Project design: involving relevant actors

The project is based on the approach 'Participatory Health Research' (Hockley et al., 2013; Wright et al., 2010). The core elements of the approach are participation, action and reflection. Approximately 40 staff (almost exclusively women) in 18 community pharmacies actively participate in the project. The project is led by the Institute of Palliative Care and Organizational Ethics at the Alpen-Adria Universität Klagenfurt, Faculty of Interdisciplinary Studies, of which the authors are members. A steering committee, consisting of Alzheimer Austria (as the umbrella organization for self-help groups), the Austrian Chamber of Pharmacists and the Institute for Palliative Care and Organizational Ethics, manages the project and takes the major decisions in the project. At certain points in the process, participation of those affected and their caregivers is enabled, e.g. in the phase of needs assessment, during workshops, in the advisory board or in the creation of a project logo. The project is being evaluated by an external evaluation.

The diverse role of community pharmacies in urban and rural settings – a user perspective

As the project takes place in two different regions in Austria, Vienna and Lower Austria, we would like to describe briefly the geographical context in order to understand better the design of the project and the methodological aspects. 'Lower Austria', one of nine provinces in Austria, is located around Vienna, Austria's capital (see Figure 10.1).

Our hypothesis was that the needs of caregivers and of people with dementia would be quite different in Vienna, the capital of Austria with 1.7 million inhabitants, and the more rural areas of Lower Austria, the biggest federal province of Austria with 1.6 million inhabitants (Statistik Austria, 2011).

The collaboration with the local self-help group Alzheimer Austria was crucial in the need-assessment phase of the project. We used a qualitative approach (Bogdan and Biklen, 2007) in the first phase of the project to gain more insight into the daily experiences of caring for a person with dementia in Vienna and Lower Austria. Another major aim was to ask caregivers about their experiences with pharmacies and especially their ideas for action in the project. Some of the results were also used to plan the contents of the workshops for the pharmacies, thus representing an action circle in this participatory health research.

We organized a focus group (Dahlin-Ivanoff and Hultberg, 2006; Krueger, 1988) in Vienna with caregivers of people with dementia using a purposeful sampling approach (Polit and Beck, 2004). Nine caregivers representing a diverse group of people with different ages, genders, number of years of caring experiences and situation of care (at home, long-term care, etc.) came together to discuss their caring-experiences, needs and ideas for the 'dementia-friendly pharmacy'. While the discussion took place, representatives of Alzheimer Austria provided care for accompanying people

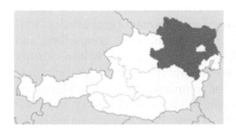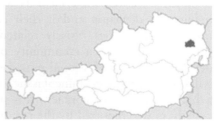

Figure 10.1 Lower Austria and Vienna

with dementia to ensure that caregivers who could not leave their relatives alone were also able to participate. Interestingly, this fact was appreciated by the caregivers, who told us afterwards that this setting enabled them to talk about topics that were rarely discussed, like the experience of violence or issues linked to sexuality.

To capture the situation in Lower Austria and to complement the topics covered in the focus group, we additionally conducted qualitative in-depth interviews with caregivers of people with dementia, again with the help of a local self-help group linked to Alzheimer Austria.

It was important to explore the experiences of caregivers from both local areas, and this led to profound insights that will be published elsewhere. One of the differences was that caregivers in Vienna stressed their 'fight against the system' with problems of bureaucracy; while caregivers in Lower Austria highlighted the lack of services for people and long distances involved in accessing available services. This difference is not surprising, considering the fact that the density of health and social services is higher in Vienna. Ideas common to both groups concerned using the pharmacy as a space for information and networking, and especially as a place to talk about dementia and to make the topic visible in the community.

Issues in caring for people living with dementia and their caregivers – the perspective of community pharmacy personnel

Based on the methodology of participatory health research outlined above, community pharmacy staff members are continuously involved in further developing the project. One important step within this approach was a needs assessment at the start of the project, where we gathered narratives on caring for people with dementia and their caregivers, and at the same time opened up a space for reflection and exchange among colleagues (Greenhalgh and Hurwitz, 1998). In the course of the project, we were systematically looking for feedback from community pharmacy staff (e.g. during workshops). Data from the external evaluation complement the findings from the narrative approach we have applied during the workshops (and results from this will be published elsewhere).

When we asked for typical as well as critical interactions with people living with dementia and/or their caregivers, community pharmacy staff raised several issues, closely related to communication, counselling and providing advice in a community pharmacy setting: they believe further development of professional practice to be important, since dementia care will become a more prominent issue for the community pharmacy. Moreover, a high frequency of contact with people living with dementia and their caregivers was reported by the majority of staff. Professional competencies related to dementia care are a key issue, and community pharmacy personnel viewed their practice with a critical eye: communicating with disoriented persons poses some challenges, as does communicating with caregivers.

On the other hand, the community pharmacy setting is believed to provide easy access to information and advice, although time constraints and lack of privacy during counselling are challenging. Moreover, community pharmacy staff view long-lasting relationships with clients as beneficial, enabling the development of trust and a deeper understanding of the daily routines of people living with dementia and their caregivers. Being able to refer caregivers in particular to counselling and support centres based on their needs is believed to be supportive, as pharmacy staff members report frequently hearing about problems related to care and to self-care during counselling. However, the majority of personnel reported a significant lack of contacts with and knowledge about support organizations. A lack of closer contacts with physicians was also mentioned, pointing to the fragmentation of the health and social care systems and a lack of systematic cooperation in Austria.

On a broader level, community pharmacy staff perceive stigmatization of dementia at a societal level to be a barrier for further engagement in dementia care, as people concerned (i.e. people living with dementia and their caregivers) may refrain from voicing their needs in the semi-public environment of a pharmacy.

When asked for key aspects that the project should ideally cover, community pharmacy staff voiced a need for a deeper understanding of dementia and issues around treatment, care and living with dementia, as well as for hands-on training in communication and in networking with other providers. In the course of the project, a need for medication management was expressed. Community pharmacy staff underlined their professional responsibility in dementia care, and a need for further development and clarification of professional roles and responsibilities.

Reorienting the community pharmacy setting and building partnerships in the community

Following up on the needs assessment of caregivers and community pharmacy staff, and building on feedback received from community pharmacy staff in the course of the project, a series of three workshops was conducted during the first phase of the project: (1) communication with those concerned and their relatives; (2) networking with support services; (3) pharmaceutical care/medication management for persons with dementia.

In the second phase of the project, the pharmacies are carrying out small-scale projects aimed at increasing the wellbeing of people with dementia and their caregivers via:

1   contributing to breaking the taboo associated with dementia by increasing visibility for issues surrounding dementia: e.g. collective activities together with community partners, such as organizing 'dementia awareness days', or activities that include people with dementia as active participants;

2   facilitating access to support services for those concerned and their caregivers, e.g. actively handing out brochures;
3   improving pharmaceutical care via counselling on medication, and initiating regular dialogue with physicians on medication issues.

These projects aimed at 'community outreach' were in their infancy at the time of publication. Community pharmacies are keen on building networks in the community. As this is not their core task, support with connecting to community-based actors enables community pharmacy staff to develop activities in their local communities. Besides this, we are working on strategies to overcome negative stereotypes associated with people living with dementia and with their caregivers, repeatedly pointing out resources and possibilities for integrating them in planning, and carrying out activities.

This project has been conceptualized as a pilot project. All experiences, material collected and approved interventions (e.g. workshop design) as well as blueprints for pharmacy-based projects will be collected to form the elements of a toolbox for a 'Dementia-friendly community pharmacy', assisting further training of community pharmacy staff and supporting sustainability.

Community pharmacies and community-based dementia care: success stories and challenges

What are the lessons learned so far during the course of the project? Below, some observations from the researchers' perspective and preliminary conclusions will be outlined, touching upon issues we consider crucial for the further development of dementia-friendly professional (i.e. health care) and community settings. As the project is still ongoing, these deliberations are tentative and will require further exploration.

Reflections on dealing with taboo and dementia in Austria

At a macro level, the historical context and the general culture in Austria have to be taken into consideration when implementing a participatory project dealing with the problems of people with dementia and their caregivers. Austrian people experienced profound and widespread trauma during the Nazi regime in the 1940s, which is not to deny that many in Austria sympathized and collaborated with the regime in that time and about 700,000 people in Austria were NSDAP members (Neugebauer, 2008), thus representing approximately 10–11 per cent of the population in 1943.

The influences of the anti-humanistic values of that period and the murder of people with disabilities and mental health problems (BIZEPS, 1996) during the years 1938–1945 cannot be underestimated. The opinion exists that common attitudes towards people with disabilities (and mental health problems or cognitive issues) in Austria in general are still burdened by the impact of this period (Naue, 2009).

Seen in this historical context at a micro level, the expressed needs of caregivers to break the taboo and talk about dementia and what it means to them is vital. This important general goal of the project was stressed repeatedly by the participating caregivers not only in the focus group and interviews but also in the advisory board of the project. The successful compensatory strategies about which they told us while caring for their relatives with dementia in the community were all linked to having talked openly about dementia, and to having explained their experiences to others in their community.

Gender aspects in participatory research with community pharmacies and people with dementia

As mentioned earlier in the text, gender aspects have an impact within the project in different regards. Working in a participatory research project, the following questions seem important and need to be reflected upon (Reitinger and Lehner, 2013): Who is participating in the project? Where and when does 'doing gender' take place? What can be observed about the collaborating field in regard to gender? These questions can be discussed at the individual, the relational and the structural levels that seem to interact in all participatory research projects.

Bearing in mind that the vast majority of the participating staff of pharmacies as well as the participating caregivers in the family are female, we can formulate hypotheses as to why this is the case. One explanation is that this represents a gendered division of labour. Gender segregation takes place vertically and horizontally within society. That means that the higher you go within a hierarchy, the more men will be in charge and that some jobs – e.g. care work – are perceived as 'female work' while others – e.g. electrical engineering – are perceived as 'male work'. In Austria gendered segregation of labour traditionally connects emphatic communication, bodywork and emotional labour with women's life and work. Additionally, this gender segregation of work leads to a devaluation of 'female' competencies (Twigg, 2006; James, 2009). The majority of professionals working in community pharmacies is also female. As the professional conception of 'being a pharmacist' was highly influenced by natural science that has changed over time, and is connected with high status, the meaning of gender segregation in this field needs further reflection and shows that a range of dimensions have to be considered (Burchell, 1996).

The concept of 'doing gender' (West and Zimmerman, 1987) helps to understand the permanent social construction processes of 'male' and 'female' in all social interactions and human practices. Within the participatory research project this can be observed and reflected, e.g. in communication processes within the steering group or the workshops. As gender relations often are interconnected with power relations – especially in participatory research projects as the one discussed here – it is interesting to see how decisions are influenced also by the gender factor. Other themes of doing gender encompass the engagement with emotions, coping with care situations in family care, or talking about communication situations in the community pharmacies.

Involving caregivers of people with dementia in service-development and community action

Collaboration with 'users' was planned at the outset of the project on two levels so that it would include the representatives of the self-help group and the caregivers themselves. We realized that it was crucial to have the possibility of direct participation of caregivers in most of the steps of the project to create a dialogue between the diverse groups, especially the pharmacy staff (not only the representatives of the chamber) and caregivers. In this chapter we speak of 'direct participation' when for example caregivers and pharmacy staff meet in person to speak for themselves.

Looking back, collaboration with the Alzheimer Austria self-help group for the needs assessment was of particular importance for the caregivers' perspectives in Vienna and Lower Austria. We decided very deliberately not to use medical services to get access to caregivers. This decision led to a group of 'empowered' caregivers, meaning that all of the participants in the needs assessment have had contact with the self-help group before and were very well aware of their needs, and could articulate them clearly. Reflecting on this fact, we found that this decision was by no means trivial, because the results showed an image of caregivers of people with dementia much at odds with what one often reads in publications. Here we had activists and people who were happy to contribute and to speak for themselves. These 'empowered caregivers' provided us with a rich understanding of their experiences and needs as a basis for further steps in the main project.

Moreover, direct participation and dialogue was made possible in the workshops with pharmacy staff, especially during a kick-off workshop for the pharmacy-based projects, where one of the caregivers was participating and giving feedback on the presentations of the individual pharmacies. This workshop was experienced as highly successful, thanks also to the direct participation of one caregiver, and again, Alzheimer Austria.

Issues related to community pharmacy practice and organization

One of the lessons learned in this project points to the development of professional roles in community pharmacy: the project has succeeded in further sensitizing community pharmacy staff to the needs of people living with dementia and their caregivers while at the same time valuing advice-giving and caring in community pharmacy. As in other sectors of society, most of the time caring is believed to be 'everyday work' going more or less unnoticed and/or mostly being defined as 'female work'. The increased sensitivity for – and recognition of – caring as an indispensable professional attitude, which manifests itself also in the organizational culture, is evidenced in the feedback voiced by community pharmacy staff during the workshops, pointing at increased confidence and empowerment when caring for people living with dementia and their caregivers.

Reflecting back on the role community pharmacies play as a local health provider is another important issue, thus encouraging the participating pharmacies to explore networking opportunities with health and social care providers: community pharmacies participating in the project show a high level of interest in networking, and have built their own local networks, e.g. with self-help groups and support organizations. Some pharmacies organize talks with providers on the pharmacy premises to publicize the providers' activities.

There are some promising steps towards including the wider community in pharmacy-based projects, e.g. one pharmacy is organizing 'dementia awareness days' in a small town supported by the mayor, and inviting such diverse actors and organizations as doctors, a photographer, support organizations and local stores to participate.

So far, the direct involvement of people living with dementia in these activities has not been realized and remains a challenge. Several possible explanations for this have already been mentioned, pointing at potential barriers at the micro (direct interaction), meso (pharmacy as a healthcare organization) and macro (societal) levels. Consistent inclusion of people living with dementia, right from the beginning of an activity, can overcome these barriers, with one example being the development of a project logo, which is described in more detail below.

The 'Dementia-friendly Community Pharmacy' logo

We consider the creation of a logo to represent the project, and be visible in the participating pharmacies as a 'model of good practice' for the participatory approach taken in the project: initiated by the steering committee of the project, a group of caregivers, pharmacists and members of the steering committee, supported by an advertising agency, held two workshops to discuss the aims of the logo and select the final design. A woman with dementia participated directly in the creative process. Because the issue of taboo and negative image of dementia and people with dementia was so strongly present in the needs assessment and narratives of all participating parties, her participation was considered especially important. One of the points discussed was whether to use the word 'dementia' in the logo, a choice that she affirmed strongly.

The logo (Figure 10.2) is thus considered as a way to make issues related to dementia visible in the pharmacies, as a prerequisite for enabling people to

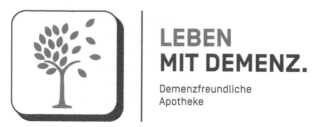

Figure 10.2 Logo 'Living with dementia. Dementia-friendly pharmacy'

asking for special services. At the same time, the logo creates visibility for the dementia-friendly pharmacies in the community.

Working in partnership: engaging community pharmacies in compassionate communities

The 'Compassionate Communities' movement in England has made a strong point of reconfiguring end of life care by 'not replacing services but enhancing, supporting and widening them' (Barry and Patel, 2013). The same holds true for reconfiguring dementia care, including end of life care in dementia. Based on the experiences gathered in dementia-friendly community pharmacies in Austria, working in partnership is believed to be effective in tapping the full potential of communities and professionals.

One of the challenges commonly known to participatory projects is the complexity and diversity of perspectives that need to be put in dialogue (von Unger, 2011). Processing the multiple perspectives of pharmacists, caregivers, self-help groups and representatives of the pharmacist chambers is highly demanding. Prior experience with transdisciplinary research in the Institute of Palliative Care and Organizational Ethics (e.g. Reitinger, 2008; Dressel et al., 2014) was an important prerequisite for the project but this had to be adapted especially because the pharmacists employ a dual logic in their work as health professionals but also as entrepreneurs. Given the complex design of this project, one of the challenges that we could not meet in the envisaged way was to include people with dementia themselves.

For future projects, we recommend including people with dementia from the very beginning, e.g. in a project's advisory board. This could not be fulfilled in our project due to various reasons, one of these being the fact that the self-help group with which we collaborated did not have any 'dementia-activists with dementia' that were easily accessible at the start of the project. This fact could also be linked to the cultural context in Austria, which has little tradition of involving 'users' in service development in general (Marent et al., 2012), and the relatively small resources that self-help groups receive from public bodies to establish structures for the involvement of users. Again, seen in the cultural context, one could say that it may still be seen as detrimental to be exposed publicly as a person with dementia, and there are very few public narratives from people with dementia in Austria.

Acknowledging and valuing the caregiving aspects of the professional role constitute an important resource, at the level of individual staff members, to engage in activities related to becoming a dementia-friendly pharmacy. However, as long as issues related to caring are (so far) not adequately recognized by professional bodies and relevant actors in health care and in education and training of pharmacy staff, these developments remain fragile. Related to this, there remains a tension between the professional and the commercial orientation in community pharmacies, in which context a balance has to be achieved.

In light of the fragmented health and social care systems, networking and integration cannot be the task of any one actor in these systems, but have to be developed in a more systematic way to support the needs of people living with dementia and their caregivers in their community. Again, as mentioned above, the participation of people with dementia and their caregivers in community pharmacy development, and generally in health and social care development, has to be valued and strengthened.

Communities and pharmacies both face opportunities and challenges when collaborating: community leaders might build on community pharmacies' resources and strengths, such as access to people living with dementia and caregivers and their mostly long-standing relationships with clients, while working on potential challenges like the lack of expertise in community-based health promotion and dementia care. Pharmacies, on the other hand, might profit from getting to know the community's capacity and existing support networks, as well as being able to link to informal networks and networking with community-based organizations, while at the same time balancing the demands of a commercial business.

In order to include the whole community in becoming 'dementia-friendly', an approach that involves community representatives (mayors, representatives from municipal offices) will be very promising. This approach is being practised in 'health-promoting villages' in some regions in Austria (including Lower Austria) and may be extended to cover issues related to dementia. Like the 'Compassionate Communities', 'health-promoting villages' have their origins in the 'Healthy Cities' movement, offering abundant experience of community-based health promotion, also focusing on older people (Reis-Klingspiegl, 2012). Relating these experiences to the findings from the 'Dementia-friendly Community Pharmacy' project might be a step worth considering in fostering the development of the afore-mentioned 'Dementia-friendly Communities' in Austria.

References

Austrian Alzheimer Society (2006) *Konsensusstatement 'Demenz' der Österreichischen Alzheimer Gesellschaft.* Update 2006. *Neuropsychiatrie* 20(4), 2010: 221–231.

Austrian Alzheimer Society (2010) *Konsensusstatement 'Demenz 2010' der Österreichischen Alzheimer Gesellschaft. Neuropsychiatrie* 24(2): 67–87.

Austrian Chamber of Pharmacists/Österreichische Apothekerkammer (ed.) (2014) *Apotheke in Zahlen 2014.* Wien.

Barry, V. and Patel, M. (2013) *An Overview of Compassionate Communities in England.* London: Murray Hall Community Trust; National Council for Palliative Care Dying Matters.

BIZEPS – Behindertenberatungszentrum – Zentrum für Selbstbestimmtes Leben (eds) (1996) Wertes unwertes Leben. Wien: [s.n.].

Blasi, Z.V., Hurley, A.C. and Volicer, L. (2002) End-of-life care in dementia: a review of problems, prospects, and solutions in practice. *Journal of the American Medical Directors Association* 3: 57–65.

Blenkinsopp, A. (2000) *Health Promotion for Pharmacists.* Oxford: Oxford University Press.

BMG Bundesministerium für Gesundheit (2011) *Frauen und Männer mit Demenz. Handlungsempfehlungen zur person-zentrierten und gendersensiblen Kommunikation für Menschen in Gesundheits- und Sozialberufen.* Edited by the Austrian Federal Ministry of Health. www.bmg.gv.at/cms/home/ attachments/6/9/4/CH1337/CMS1316599156685/iff_bmg_demenz-folder_ barr_14_9_2011.pdf (accessed 10 October 2014).

BMG Bundesministerium für Gesundheit (2013) *Geschlechtersensibel werden. Nachdenken über Gender im Umgang mit Menschen mit Demenz. Eine Handreichung für Gesundheits- und Sozialberufe.* Edited by the Austrian Federal Ministry of Health. www.bmg.gv.at/cms/home/attachments/6/9/4/CH1337/ CMS1316599156685/demenz_geschlechtersensibel_werden_0fehler.pdf (accessed 10 October 2014).

Bogdan, R.C. and Biklen, S.K. (2007) *Qualitative Research for Education. An Introduction to Theories and Methods.* Boston, MA: Pearson Allyn & Bacon.

Burchell, B.J. (1996) Gender segregation, size of workplace and the public sector. *Gender, Work & Organization* 3: 227–235.

Dahlin-Ivanoff, S. and Hultberg, J. (2006) Understanding the multiple realities of everyday life: basic assumptions in focus-group methodology. *Scandinavian Journal of Occupational Therapy* 13: 125–132.

Dressel, G., Berger W., Heimerl K. and Winiwarter V. (eds) (2014) *Interdisziplinär und transdisziplinär forschen. Praktiken und Methoden.* Bielefeld: transcript.

Greenhalgh, T. and Hurwitz, B. (1998) *Narrative-based Medicine.* London: BMJ Books.

Gröning, K. and Heimerl, K. (2012) *Menschen mit Demenz in der Familie. Ethische Prinzipien im täglichen Umgang.* Wien: Picus.

Haslbeck, J.W. and Schaeffer, D. (2009) Routines in medication management: the perspective of people with chronic conditions. *Chronic Illness* 5(3): 184–196.

Hockley, J.M., Froggatt, K. and Heimerl, K. (2013) *Participatory Research in Palliative Care: Actions and Reflections.* Oxford: Oxford University Press.

James, V. (2009) Positioning emotion through the body and bodywork: a reflection through nursing as craft. *International Journal of Work Organisation and Emotion* 3(2): 146–160.

Kellehear, A. (2005) *Compassionate Cities: Public Health and End-of-Life Care.* London: Routledge.

Kellehear, A. (2009) Dementia and dying: the need for a systematic policy approach. *Critical Social Policy* 29 1): 146–157.

Kojer, M. and Schmidl, M. (eds) (2011) *Demenz und Palliative Geriatrie in der Praxis. Heilsame Betreuung unheilbar demenzkranker Menschen.* Wien: Springer.

Krueger, R. (1988) *Focus Groups: A Practical Guide for Applied Research.* Thousand Oaks, CA: Sage.

Marent, B., Forster, R. and Nowak, P. (2012) Theorizing participation in health promotion: a literature review. *Social Theory & Health* 10: 188–207.

Naue, U. (2009) Österreichische Behindertenpolitik im Kontext nationaler Politik und internationaler Diskurse zu Behinderung. *SWS – Rundschau* 49(3): 274–292.

Neugebauer, W. (2008) *Der österreichische Widerstand 1938–1945.* Wien: Edition Steinbauer.

NICE/SCIE (2006) *Dementia: Supporting People with Dementia and Their Carers in Health and Social Care.* NICE Guidelines. London: National Institute for Health and Care Excellence/Social Care Institute for Excellence. www.nice.org.uk/guidance/CG042/chapter/Key-priorities-for-implementation

Polit, D.F. and Beck, C.T. (2004) *Nursing Research: Principles and methods.* Philadelphia, PA: Lippincott Williams & Wilkins.

Reis-Klingspiegl, K. (2012) Lebenswerte Lebenswelten in einer Geografie des Alterns. Partizipation, Mobilität und Autonomie in ländlichen Räumen in der Steiermark. In: Kümpers, S. and Heusinger, J. (eds) *Autonomie trotz Armut und Pflegebedarf?: Altern unter Bedingungen von Marginalisierung.* Bern: H. Huber.

Reitinger, E. (2008) *Transdisziplinäre Praxis: Forschen im Sozial- und Gesundheitswesen.* Heidelberg: Systemische Forschung im Carl-Auer-Verlag.

Reitinger, E. and Lehner, E. (2013) Gender perspectives in Austrian participatory research in palliative care for older people. In: Hockley, J. Froggatt, K. and Heimerl, K. (eds) *Participatory Research in Palliative Care. Actions and Reflections.* Oxford: Oxford University Press, pp. 138–148.

Small, N., Froggatt, K. and Downs, M. (2008) *Living and Dying with Dementia: Dialogues about Palliative Care.* Oxford: Oxford University Press.

Statistik Austria (2011) *Volkszählungen, Registerzählung, Abgestimmte Erwerbsstatistik.* www.statistik.at/web_de/statistiken/bevoelkerung/volkszaehlungen_registerzaehlungen_abgestimmte_erwerbsstatistik/index.html

Twigg, J. (2006) *The Body in Health and Social Care.* Basingstoke: Palgrave Macmillan.

von Unger, H. (2011) Partizipative Gesundheitsforschung: Wer partizipiert woran? Participatory Health Research: Who Participates in What? Investigación participativa en salud: ¿Quién participa en qué? *FQS: Forum: Qualitative Social Research Sozialforschung* 1(7). Retrieved from: www.qualitative-research.net

West, C. and Zimmerman, D.H. (1987) Doing gender. *Gender & Society* 2(1): 125–151.

Wißmann, P. and Gronemeyer, R. (2008) *Demenz und Zivilgesellschaft – eine Streitschrift.* Frankfurt a. M.: Mabuse.

World Health Organization, Welfare Canada (1986) *Ottawa Charter for Health Promotion (Charte d'Ottowa pour la promotion de la santé)*. Ottawa: WHO. www.euro.who.int/__data/assets/pdf_file/0004/129532/Ottawa_Charter.pdf?ua=1 (accessed 10 October 2014).

Wright, M.T., Gardner, B., Roche, B., von Unger, H. and Ainlay, C. (2010) Building an international collaboration on participatory health research. *Progress in Community Health Partnerships: Research, Education, and Action* 4(1): 31–36.

11 A convent initiative

Compassionate Community in Solothurn, Switzerland

Elisabeth Wappelshammer and
Christine Weissenberg

Pre-professional forms of a supportive culture of care include competences that are at risk of going unnoticed. To answer the care needs of very old, frail and dying people, it is important to raise awareness of this kind of knowledge in order to develop integrated care models.

Where in our economised society are there models from which society can learn? A highly traditional model of caring is based on the monastic tradition, upon which we focused within the participatory research project, 'A Municipal Culture of Care: The Caring Community in Life and Death'. We combined the findings with the local and regional discourses of professional experts in care and medical treatment.

Similarly to other convents, the ageing community of the contemplative convent 'Namen Jesu' has succeeded in a striking manner in coping without professional help for many years. Our approach follows the thesis that relevant factors can be utilised for other actors in the care setting.

Beginning with an enquiry into coping strategies within the ageing community, the project aims at translating the findings into professional structures of old-age care as well as into civil–social structures. Our thesis is as follows: the successful integration of relevant aspects of our results within the discourses of long-term and ambulant nursing as well as in the culture of civil society, could mean that the culture of care changes in an innovative way.

Likewise, it must be assumed that traditional life in a convent cannot simply be replicated. Its origin is bound to special historical contexts, and social modernisation has also changed life within the convent walls. The value of insights from investigating the monastic tradition largely relates to the unfamiliar perspective regarding hitherto unquestioned aspects of current practice in treatment and care (Kreutzer, 2011: 254).

The project in the national context of palliative care

According to our understanding, rather similar discourses take place in Switzerland as they do throughout the European context as a whole concerning palliative care. Here, too, professional health and care systems are reaching their limits in terms of caring for old, chronically ill and dying people:

- Services regarding hospice and palliative care are not yet reaching all those people who have need of them (Bundesamt für Gesundheit, 2012: 4). A representative survey by the Federal Office for Health (Bundesamt für Gesundheit, 2009) showed that 44 per cent of the participants would make use of palliative care in case of incurable illness, if this option were available. The vast majority (91 per cent) of the participants believed that palliative care should be available to all severely ill and dying people.
- Some 75 per cent of the population would like to be able to die at home, yet more than 80 per cent are still dying in hospital or in long-term nursing homes. In fact, only 20 per cent of people die at home (with considerable regional differencies) or in another similar place.
- With rising life expectancy, the majority of people die after a long illness and phase of nursing, meaning that the demand for nursing and care is also rising (Bundesamt für Gesundheit, 2009: 3). Depending on predicted trends, the number of 80-year-old and older people living in Switzerland will rise from about 450,000 people presently to about 1,156,000 people by 2060 (Bundesamt für Statistik, 2013: 3). Last, but not least, the babyboomer generation will be reaching the final stage of life in the coming decades (Eychmüller and Cina, 2010: 221).
- A considerable proportion (approximately 60 per cent) of the population is cared for at home by informal caregivers, of whom about two-thirds are women and one-third are men, having an average age of about 66 years (Perrig-Chiello et al., 2010: 23). The outpatient and community-based care requirements for patients and caregivers increase significantly.

National palliative care plan

In 2009, Switzerland's health officials started a national strategy of palliative care, with a plan to run until 2015. The main objective is to achieve the widespread establishment of the palliative care concept and practice in Swiss society. The report and forward plan of the national strategy 2012–2015 in particular contain the observation that the number of annual deaths is increasing steadily and that care during the final phase of life is becoming ever more complex, not only medically, but also concerning psychological and spiritual needs. Moreover ageing populations increasingly desire a degree of autonomy and participation in medical treatment and nursing care.

Our project is dedicated to the framework of the national palliative care strategy plan – in particular at the level of cantons and local communities. Our participatory research approach includes the target groups of professional and voluntary experts at cantonal and local level. Moreover, a special focus concerns the ageing community of a convent.

Critique of biomechanics-dominated approaches and the rationing of resources

Increasing critique can be observed in expert discourse, which requires a broadening of themes beyond pure medical questions regarding end-of-life care.

> Here it becomes clear that issues at the end of life concern far more than pure medical or nursing competence according to the current, rather biomechanical definition. If the spectrum of subjects is limited, as the high number of deaths in hospitals and long-term nursing homes suggests, then great unease seems to arise.
>
> (Eychmüller and Cina, 2010: 221)

This type of unease was confirmed by most of our interview partners who work as health professionals. Furthermore, they described what would actually be required: 'Certainly the best treatment of pain and other forms of suffering are a mutual partnership-based and respectful form of decision-making. This requires time, tranquillity, talks and preferably a clear head' (Eychmüller and Cina[1], 2010: 221).

In particular, the limiting of care options in terms of 'end-of-life care' is perceived very critically where palliative care for people with long-term disease is concerned:

> The point is that now the health insurance, or at least Santé Suisse, actually only wishes to finance end-of-life care. This now opens yet another interface. And we run quite a high risk of falling between two stools again, because we actually undertake palliative care. So, this is at the moment my focus within the palliative care network, that we emphasise palliative care and not end-of-life care, because the concept of end-of-life care starts too late for us. Now we have taken part in a pilot project, involving both our quality management and our performance measurement tool. Meanwhile, the insurers only want to pay for end-of-life care. In fact, they do not notice us, because end-of-life care is performed only for a matter of some months at the most. The work of an institution is only recorded if it does not last longer than 6 months until a person dies. What happens outside this timeframe is not regarded as end-of-life care. These are issues which weigh upon me very strongly. But we undertake palliative care in the truest sense of the word from morning to evening. And from my point of view this should actually be the issue. And finally there is again the problem of over-professionalisation. It becomes technical again, new terminology is created again, and the human being is forgotten, always, always, always, always.
>
> (Interview Graf, lines 160–177)

In Switzerland, assisted suicide is not a punishable offence, and is largely undertaken by organisations such as Dignitas and Exit. Within palliative care, this development is perceived and commented upon in very critical terms and is linked to the trend towards economisation and the dominance of cost-intensive medicine as well as the expense associated with nursing and care services:

> The discussion surrounding assisted suicide seems to be a symptom for this unease, and in debates about costs, the issue of 'rationing' is always flashing up furtively. Here the issue should be more about the quality of medical indications and medical interventions at the end of life and less about the costs: A course of radiotherapy or a new stent within the last weeks of life are paid for by insurers without questioning the objectives or 'expected clinical benefit'. Care at home with auxiliary services and basic care provision is partly paid from the person's own private resources.
> (Eychmüller and Cina, 2010: 221)

The management of a regional nursing home expressed a critical view of the tendency by health insurers to sometimes finance poor quality care and provided the following example: 'Treatment for a decubitus is paid for, but not the prophylaxis to prevent it occurring, which is rather care-intensive' (Interview Mathys, lines 16–23).

General situation in convents

As can also be seen in the Namen Jesu convent, monasteries and convents saw their last waves of entry during the 1950s and 1960s. This means that the scope of traditional monastic forms of living is decreasing, the communities are ageing and increasingly facing difficult decisions regarding the care of their frail brothers and sisters. Often the future of communities and their buildings is unclear, and old age is a central concern. The care that is required often cannot be performed any longer by the community itself and, in such cases, professional experts must be employed:

> In the convents the 'nursing need of the sisters' must be looked at anew … Through the changes in the age structure, the situation has changed drastically. We cannot carry out the care of our own sisters anymore. For many years we have had to recruit caregivers from outside. That means our care-dependent sisters are not cared for by their own community, which has led of course to big changes, both structurally and personally. There is not the usual family concern any more, the conditions of public health services must be fulfilled, etc.
> This is a great challenge for the persons responsible of the cloister. Architectural, financial and structural questions must be discussed and managed anew. The challenge now is: On one hand the care-dependent

are concerned by this development, on the other hand, it also needs big efforts, for instance in-house training, so that the staff can understand how the structure of a convent works and can accept the traditions here. They must be aware that the nursing home is the home of the sisters

(Interview Juchli, lines 20–36)

A professional part-time nurse has also been employed in the Namen Jesu convent. Her integration in the everyday life of the convent has not been easy for both sides, because of contradictory expectations to some extent. On the nuns' side a completely new kind of leadership is required, with high levels of transparency, while the professional care service provider is faced with a culture based on historically acquired rules of strict discretion and partly on highly individual habits – far from any standards of quality management in professionalised geriatric care and nursing. For both sides, this can be very confusing and may cause real conflicts.

Monastic building structures are often many centuries old. In the case of the Namen Jesu convent there is much evidence of how little the architecture is appropriate for persons in old age, especially if measured against the norms and standards of geriatric care. Even if two lifts are installed, stairs and steps remain obstacles that are not manageable for all nuns or that at the least represent an athletic challenge. Yet this architecture constitutes the home environment for the members of the convent and guarantees continuity of time and social environment.

Visions of change need unexpected and unfamiliar effects

Experiences with death and loss are inevitable. Public health discourses increasingly demand that this central field of human experience is given a central place in society (Kellehear, 2005). The challenge is to develop communities in which social cooperation and mutual responsibility are performed, with care provided both for the vulnerable dying and for those who care for them, and later mourn them. Adequate visions of change in the sense of a society in which a culture of care is regarded as centrally important are both challenging and complex – in particular connected to local and regional development of a culture of compassion and political concepts of care culture beyond standardisation and professionalisation. Which existing communities, however, can provide us with relevant examples?

In the Swiss convent Namen Jesu, we were able to make observations, carry out interviews and hold two workshops. After all, here too, death is visible. Slowly but inevitably even the model of cloister life is dying. Nevertheless, significant differences to other institutions can be observed. Illness and deficits in health terms seem to be not so dominant as in other settings. On the contrary, growing old seems to succeed with a great degree of *grandezza*, with or without dementia: 'Aging with Grace', as David Snowdon (2002) expresses it.

This was, in any case, the most surprising aspect of our observations; and astonishment and surprise seem to us actually to be rather beneficial effects, which can help find a way out from all too restrictive dynamics. In a situation in which most representatives of relevant professions and leaderships of administrative and political departments feel very much restricted by the current logics of care, which themselves hinder the formulation of desires for change and renewal, it is worthwhile to use perspectives that can offer the 'shock of the new'. The perspective of monastic life can achieve such impacts because the world behind cloister walls is shaped by a special mixture of old traditions and modern influence, in which the trends towards economisation, professionalisation and specialisation do not yet have so much influence as they do outside. Thus this form of care culture may be able to serve to open the door for generally required steps towards change that can put care at the heart of society.

Development of the project

In the Name Jesu convent in Solothurn, largely self-directed care is undertaken in impressive fashion by the community itself. The elderly and very old nuns have managed extensively to cope without professional help and care up until now. For a long time a part-time cook has been the only professional nurse, albeit with another job description – helping with the cooking and building up confidence through working together. Everyday life is characterised by remarkable autonomy and dignity. But life has also become fragile, with the sisters increasingly needing help from outside. However, what happens when pre-professional and professional care encounter one another? Which care approaches used by the ageing community should be retained? What can professionals learn from this?

Triangulation of methods

In terms of a productive connection between participatory research and theoretical discourse we focus on the question of which relevant aspects of discourses in palliative care can be identified in this kind of religious and spiritual community.

We describe the results of qualitative investigations by means of observations, interviews and workshops inside and outside the convent. Triangulation of methods was suitable for avoiding possible blind spots in our findings. Above all, participant observations helped in understanding aspects of monastic care culture, beyond the reflection of everyday culture in the interviews. In total, we carried out 13 interviews within the convent itself and within the setting of the Swiss convents and 16 qualitative interviews with professionals. Experts of professional care or medical treatment were also asked questions about their view of convents, as far as participants were familiar with them. In addition we conducted a workshop about the internal view of the convent and an interdisciplinary workshop with representatives of the convent, different professions and politicians as well as voluntary services.

Challenges and learning effects

During the process of research in the convent we faced particular challenges:

- The first challenge was to establish the project in the convent altogether. The convent belongs to a contemplative community, the Capuchins, where silence and spirituality are regarded as central values. We assume that we only succeeded in establishing the project by taking part in the everyday life of the community, which gave us the opportunity to carry out participant observation and build necessary trust among the participants.
- The involvement with the monastic community, created by our integration in everyday life there, led to another great challenge. The growing needs of the community make it tempting for those coming from outside to interfere or even take on leading roles in some respects, as became clear while talking to some of our interview partners. We also had to realise through the example of the installation of a chair lift that we too were not free of this desire to help out in the context of convent life.
- Finally, it is necessary to understand modernisation in the context of cloister life – with principles like individualism and pluralism – just as we find it generally in society. The current model of convent life only in part reflects aspects of the original form of spiritual communities. Especially since the Second Vatican Council in the 1960s, reforms have taken place, and thus generalising about 'convent life' requires a differentiated understanding.

Results

Coping strategies of the convent community

The following text introduces the life of a special community of a convent and its successful coping strategies from the viewpoint of living and dying in old age. In the analysis of the results of observations, interviews and workshops we combine our findings with analyses of Joan Tronto (2013) concerning a fundamental change, shifting care into the centre of society. How do coping strategies of this ageing community distinguish themselves from the perspective of the political scientist Joan Tronto? What would she perhaps perceive on a visit to the convent community?

Perspectives of carers and those being cared for

In democratic settings, both carers as well as those being cared for are involved. According to their area of competence, everyone takes part in the care culture.

In accordance with their vows upon joining the order, the nuns of the convent experience a fundamental attachment to each other, which goes far beyond personal sympathy. This determines mutual loyalty in everyday life, even if conflicts occur. The convent cannot be easily identified as a democratic setting, because beside democratic facilities, such as voting for the head of the convent and the debates in the council of the convent, the traditional culture of the cloister is characterised by a strong hierarchy based on the principle of obedience. Nevertheless, it seems that everybody is integrated on an equal basis into this community of care. Even if women themselves are ill and in need of care, they participate in the care of other sisters, if only through small gestures of support. Therefore it can be perceived that a nun who has fallen ill with dementia helps another sister who is mentally healthy but has physical problems using the stairs to the refectory. Above all everybody perceives the others as 'sisters' and it is clear that everybody has needs to care for, even those whose task primarily is caring. 'Human dignity happens when I am a human being to a human being, if I am a sister to the sister, respectively if the sister is a sister to the sister' (Interview Juchli, lines 300–302).

Relational autonomy and dignity

At 94 years old, Sister Hildegard (pseudonym) is the oldest member of the convent and suffers from severe heart failure. However, she still maintains her position as convent custodian on a daily basis, refusing to give up this social role. She takes pleasure in using her 'Trottinette' (a push-along scooter) to travel the long corridors and laughs mischievously when others find her going along at full tilt, steering with one hand while holding her walking stick to push forward in the other.

Sisterhood seems to promote both relational dignity and relational autonomy. In the concept of relational autonomy, neither the dependence and autonomy of those who are in need of care nor that of their carers are ignored. Both are autonomous as well as dependent. 'Dignity is socially constructed, individually perceived, embodied and relational' (Pleschberger, 2005: 37).

In convents, public life and privacy are complementary spheres, which nurture the dignity of community members as a manifestation of social life. Several times during each day, the nuns celebrate a (semi-) public life with one another, which serves a higher communal purpose and at times also incorporates guests from outside. At the same time, the option also exists for convent members to be able to withdraw into the intimate sphere of the closed community and their single cells.

In this culture, a highly beneficial balance is achieved between (semi-) public participation in the ritual phases of the day as well as experiences of community at work, spare time and meals on the one hand and intimate retreat on the other hand, as stipulated in the discourse around dignity in terms of 'acknowledgment' and relational dignity (Pleschberger, 2005: 28ff. and 113ff.). The everyday experience of the value of this balance means that the neoliberal idea that public care could be a danger for the whole community simply does not apply (Tronto, 2013: 144).

It seems that mutual care within the convent never intervenes further into the personal sphere than the community regards as necessary. Here care is regarded as serving an autonomous lifestyle, whereas forms of care that give those cared for the feeling that they are helpless are avoided.

The culture of 'sisterhood' means that the care culture also diverges from dyadic nursing arrangements, which generally dominate in the family context. Joan Tronto identifies dangers of caring dyads becoming an 'uncompassionate hierarchy', and she suggests that it is important to address the possibilities of a 'triangulation' of care (Tronto, 2013: 153). Even if a relationship between two persons involved in care does develop, in the convent there remains at least one other person responsible for the area of health care as a whole or other sisters may intervene where required, and there is now also a professional nurse from outside the convent. Thus the convent seems to be a place where the possibilities for 'triangulation' are more easily available than in families.

On the production of 'others' – the cycle inspired by neoliberalism

A central aspect of political care culture is the neoliberal trend to produce 'others', whose apparent inability to assert themselves economically is interpreted as a decline of their personal value. As a result, annoyance, frustration and mistrust are nurtured on a wide basis, complemented by forms of political control and sanction (Tronto, 2013: 145). In such a culture, no broadly conceived culture of mutual care can develop. Neoliberal politics tends to produce a loss of personal value where there is a perceived lack of the appropriate success in terms of economy and consumption.

The nuns of the convent community have consciously decided to be 'others'. From the outset, the life of the relatively poor community is based upon embracing poverty and remains far away from the logic of the neoliberal economic system, which generates more and more needs together with social status, devaluation and exclusion. At the same time, a huge capacity for enjoyment can be observed in the everyday life of the nuns, which probably acts as the most effective cultural barrier against neoliberal dynamics.

Inspiring networks beyond cloister walls

Although high and ancient stone walls surround the convent, various levels of contact with the larger community of the town and its citizens may be observed.

One of the key experiences during our research in Solothurn – both within as well as outside the cloister community – was that the concept of a 'culture of care' represents an inspiring catalyst for discourse within the relevant professional fields.

Nuns, volunteers and professionals who were active in the areas of outpatient, long-term and medical care embraced this concept. In the first instance it was professionals in particular who used it to articulate their critique of phenomena such as economisation, professionalisation and standardisation, which were seen as problematic issues. Despite or maybe because of the fact that the term is not clearly defined, it is capable of inspiring various actors to consider new perspectives and to express things for which the words were apparently lacking up to now.

Care culture: connections between convent, professional services and facilities, representatives of civil society, social administration and politics

How might the care culture of the convent ultimately provide inspiration for the world outside? One established connection concerns the local involvement of citizens who feel linked to the convent community. They understand the lives of 'others' and feel a sense of personal attachment to the community.

Regardless of life within the convent, society has need of a culture of care which is based on the autonomy and dignity of every single person and offers the chance to participate actively, particularly during the last phase of life. The experiences of the Namen Jesu convent reveal a very old form of caring for one another in which strengthening the ability to care for oneself holds important value. This form of care deserves to receive attention in other social areas too and also from the organisations of social and health care systems, which still retain a paternalistic approach today.

In recognition of this, our research concentrated not only upon the convent, but included other stakeholders within the municipality and the canton of Solothurn: Doctors, in particular the founder of the cantonal palliative care network, the cantonal health department, an organisation providing outpatient care, a dementia-nursing centre, a hospice association, an outpatient service providing support for families caring for people with disabilities, outpatient hospice care, a canton-wide platform for volunteer work, a neighbourhood association, and last but not least, politicians.

In a situation in which most representatives of relevant professions, administrative and political departments feel severely restricted by operational logics, which themselves hinder the formulation of wishes for change and renewal, it is worthwhile to make use of all perspectives that offer 'the shock of the new'. The convent Namen Jesu is able to provide such effects, because most of the nuns in the community are old and very old women and are often already so frail that one is surprised as an outsider that the community is still able to manage everyday life. Likewise every single one of the nuns exhibits a rather special, sometimes even wayward, form of autonomy and dignity. Especially impressive, however, is the way in which the cloister community deals with the resources, enabling them to also provide a service to people outside the convent, e.g. to women going through difficult phases of life. This creates a reciprocity of care, which is rarely observed in inpatient facilities for medical and nursing care.

However, those who are aware of the special complexity of this small monastic '*oikos*' are thus also inspired to have their own thoughts about, for example, the establishment of a 'new care culture', outlined as a bottom-up strategy of a community-oriented life based on the idea of neighbourhood. Short-, medium- and long-term aims include, for example, care culture as a component of medical training at university as well as in school curricula and raising public awareness within the local community by stakeholders – also in the sense of the principle of 'sister- and brotherhood' as a quality of a new care culture. Finally, the everyday life of the convent provides inspiration in terms of the rituals that permeate daily life, which contrast with the post-modern phenomena of growing alienation in spatial and temporal terms (cf. Rosa, 2013: 139ff.).

It was and is entirely clear to our partners in this participatory research process that the monastic tradition could not be transposed completely into other organisational settings, and even the nuns themselves regard such an idea either as inadequate or antiquated. But awareness and imagination are inspired to use central principles of this kind of centries-old explicit and implicit knowledge to benefit a contemporary culture of care – for example, concerning a good life in autonomy and dignity even as a very old and frail person.

Both the nuns who joined the final interdisciplinary and transdisciplinary workshop and the convent, as the location for this event, thus served as catalysts for new conceptual links concerning the local and regional structure of care and nursing and above all for a lively and fluid discourse. In this respect, one participant in the workshop coming from the medical sector commented on the role of religious communities as follows: 'These organisations are "infectious" and inspiring' (Cina, workshop report of comments, p. 6).

Summary and outlook

As a first step, observations, interviews and a workshop were carried out within the convent, to determine the culture of care among a group of ageing nuns. In the second step, the local and regional potential of a new culture of care beyond the convent community was investigated with the help of interviews. In a joint workshop with all target groups, professionals and representatives of voluntary organisations, further ideas for the culture of care were developed, which can make a contribution to establishing principles of a new care culture based on solidarity with others.

In this way, the project generated comprehensive data, which are still available for further analysis regarding various themes. Likewise the participatory approach of the research facilitated the development of a network of interested experts together with members of the community at local and regional level. This network could be activated in a subsequent project to continue, intensify and widen the discourse about a new culture of care.

Note

1   Christoph Cina was one of our interview partners.

References

Bundesamt für Gesundheit BAG/Schweizerische Konferenz der kantonalen Gesundheitsdirektorinnen und –direktoren (GDK) (2009) *Nationale Strategie Palliative Care 2010–2012*, Bern.
Bundesamt für Gesundheit BAG/Schweizerische Konferenz der kantonalen Gesundheitsdirektorinnen und –direktoren (GDK) (2012) *Nationale Strategie Palliative Care 2012–2015*, Bern.
Bundesamt für Statistik/BFS (2013) *Zukünftige Bevölkerungsentwicklung.*
Eychmüller, S. and Cina, C. (2010) Licht im Dunkel für die letzte Lebensphase –was bietet Palliative Care? *PrimaryCare* 10(12): 221–222.
Kellehear, A. (2005) *Compassionate Cities. Public Health and End-of-Life Care.* New York: Routledge.
Kreutzer, S. (2011) Glaube als biographischer Rückhalt im Umgang mit Krankheit und Sterben. In: H. Remmers (ed.) *Pflegewissenschaft im interdisziplinären Dialog. Eine Forschungsbilanz.* V&R unipress, Universitätsverlag Osnabrück, S. 239–257.
Perrig-Chiello, P., Höpflinger, F. and Schnegg, B. (2010) *Pflegende Angehörige von älteren Menschen in der Schweiz.* Schlussbericht: SwissAgeCare.
Pleschberger, S. (2005) *Nur nicht zur Last fallen. Sterben in Würde aus der Sicht alter Menschen in Pflegeheimen.* Freiburg i. B.: Lambertus.
Rosa, H. (2013) *Beschleunigung und Entfremdung.* Frankfurt a.M.: Suhrkamp.
Snowdon, D. (2002) *Aging with Grace. What the Nun Study Teaches Us about Leading Longer, Healthier, and More Meaningful Lives.* New York: Bantam Books.
Tronto, J.C. (2013) *Caring Democracy. Markets, Equality and Justice.* New York: New York University Press.

12 Community palliative care in Eastern Switzerland

The role of local forums in developing palliative care culture and enabling ethical discourse

Katharina Linsi and Karin Kaspers-Elekes

Introduction

> The Federal state and the cantons anchor palliative care together with the key actors in the health sector and other areas. Critically ill and dying persons in Switzerland thus receive a palliative care that is adapted to their needs, improving their quality of life.

With these words, Switzerland's healthcare policy formulated the major goals of the 'National Palliative Care Strategy' in Switzerland (Bundesamt für Gesundheit – BAG, 2013). One aim in particular with regard to Swiss citizens and dying stands in the foreground: in a representative survey of the population, three-quarters of those who participated said they would prefer to die 'at home' (GfK Switzerland AG, 2010). To do justice to this desire to have access to palliative care near one's home, an organizational form that would enable this needs to be identified.

Eastern Switzerland is among the regions in which palliative care is relatively well developed. 'Even in this favourable situation, community palliative care is still long way from being standard care at the end of life' (Eychmüller and Domeisen, 2013). In the model presented here, we adopt the positive starting point in Eastern Switzerland and seek answers to the question of how the wish of citizens to die at home might be fulfilled and a community-based palliative care service developed.

Resources for the development of community-based palliative care: the *'palliative ostschweiz'* association

The *palliative ostschweiz* (Palliative Eastern Switzerland) association works to promote the further development of palliative care both at cantonal level and nationally as a regional association within palliative.ch. The *palliative ostschweiz* association has the object of improving access to palliative care for all those living in the regional area.[1] To this end, it promotes understanding of and provides information about palliative care to all professional sectors within health care and social policy, the general public, politicians and administrative bodies. *Palliative ostschweiz* provides resources for the designing of regional concepts for needs-oriented planning and to support those with an interest in the development of palliative care services. This also includes building networks between specialists, voluntary groups, organizations and institutions with the aim of steering the further development of the palliative care landscape, as well as communicating information about this to the general public.

Building networks as a core activity

In the course of developing palliative support, *local network building* has proven to be a valuable prerequisite for needs-oriented palliative care provision. The *palliative ostschweiz* association thus brings specialists from different organizations and professions from within the region engaged in palliative care together in networks. An inter-professional approach, which is based on mutual recognition and appreciation, is a key prerequisite for the complex requirements and challenges regarding which persons with illnesses requiring palliative care should experience such support. In this context, particular emphasis is laid upon voluntary organizations.

Research study: 'network organization' as a core competence

Inspired by the Kerala model of 'neighbourhood network palliative care' (Kumar, 2007) a team of researchers at the Palliative Care Centre in St. Gallen initiated a community-based palliative care project in three regions in North-Eastern Switzerland and in Liechtenstein. The goal of the study was to prepare communities for active participation in end-of-life care. The project brought together professionals, volunteers and community leaders to develop a community palliative care programme (cf. Eychmüller and Domeisen, 2013: 76).

The study began by addressing two questions: the status quo of care for critically ill and dying persons within Eastern Switzerland and in the Principality of Liechtenstein (the catchment area of *palliative ostschweiz*) should be surveyed and the question addressed of whether existing regional care services constitute an adequate network capable of enabling persons the option of dying at home (*Palliative Care in der Gemeinde*, handbook, Palliativzentrum Kantonsspital St. Gallen, undated). Although most Swiss citizens wish to die at home, the reality is somewhat different: most people currently die in homes for the elderly or care homes or in hospital. In 2009, 62,500 people died in Switzerland, of whom 25,300 (41 per cent) died in hospital and 24,800 (40 per cent) in care homes or homes for the elderly, while 12,300 persons (20 per cent) died at home or at another location (BFS, 2009).

Four key goals were defined, in the achievement of which palliative care should play a helpful role: self-help, self-determination, security and support. Along with management of symptoms, decision-making and the support of close relatives, network organization is required. Based on the experiences of the St. Gallen palliative care centre, 'Network organization for care at home' was defined as *one* core competence that is required if these four goals are to be achieved.

A local palliative care network is understood as one that brings together people and organizations for the care of critically ill and dying persons at home (Palliativzentrum Kantonsspital St. Gallen, undated: 4). The creation of such a network enables the scope for individually tailored solutions to be expanded at the organizational and individual level. At the same time, cooperation becomes the norm – to the benefit of the affected persons requiring palliative support.

The results of the research study and experiences gathered in the course of the research period have led to a series of recommendations for practical application, published in the handbook *Palliative Care in der Gemeinde* (Palliativzentrum Kantonsspital St. Gallen, undated). These include 'recommendations for the creation of a core group within the community' with a common identity, a 'Palliative Care Forum'. The guidelines set out here have flowed into the practical implementation in Eastern Switzerland as described in this chapter, and they continue to exert considerable influence on this today.

Palliative care forums

Practical experience shows that the creation of an interdisciplinary working group requires the involvement of at least one organization that is recognized and established in the primary palliative care sector within the region to drive this development. In accordance with Cicely Saunders's (1984) concept of 'total pain', this working group should ideally include representatives of medical services and nursing care, together with those providing psychosocial and spiritual support. The core group invites a range of potential and essential workers and organizations, e.g. an organization involved in outpatient care (known in Switzerland as 'Spitex'). In addition, it is desirable to have the 'transitions' to specialized palliative care in mind when building networks. Thus local networks arise, referred to as the 'palliative care forums', that are central to community-based palliative care. These are important organizational units for developing, designing and embedding palliative care in local communities and regions. The document that sets out the guidelines for their functions defines such forums as follows:

This, the smallest cell in the body of palliative care in Eastern Switzerland, represents a logical, manageable and functionally collaborative organizational unit. The precise scope is not defined.[2]

The forum thus developed utilizes existing structures in order to keep organization as simple as possible. It comprises all important network partners within primary palliative care (as a minimum, Spitex, general practitioners and pastoral care), while at the same time integrating local political actors. The forum works closely together with the providers of specialist palliative care, ideally including these as constituent members of the forum.

Involving the local community has a particular value where the development of a forum is concerned. It is desirable that the local authorities function as the forum's commissioning body and make resources available – even if these are relatively limited – such as help with publicity or venues for meeting.

Participatory development of a local palliative care concept

Using the participatory model, the forum facilitates the joint development of the palliative care concept. Through the discussion process, connective relationships, local care culture and a fundamental ethical approach are strengthened. This creates the basis for concrete implementation of regional palliative care, allows dependencies and conflicting values to be discussed, and in the process develops a 'common language' and lays the foundation for a respectful approach to working together with others. A culture of communication and cooperation evolves. On this basis, the palliative care concept regulates cooperation between the individual partners in the forum, delineates responsibilities and makes both internal and external networks visible. Quality assurance and optimization take place through the networking of existing structures and closing gaps in services. The provision of information to political actors and the general public in the area served by the forum is a key component here.

The forums are supported by the umbrella organization *palliative ostschweiz*, with the forums being in legal and financial terms constituent parts of this body. They have clearly defined catchment areas, which correspond to the service areas of outpatient care services. To date, nine forums have been set up in the region.

A stepwise approach to founding a palliative care forum

The Am Alten Rhein (AAR) forum is used as an example here to describe the steps required to facilitate the creation of a resilient local network structure and culture. The steps are outlined in this section.

Step 1: Clarifying the mandate

For the successful creation of a forum, a mandate is indispensable. Whether this mandate comes 'from above' or at the initiative of groups or individuals is not important. What is important is that an official and clear mandate is produced as a result.

As the initiator of community-based palliative care forums, a part of the mandate comes from *palliative ostschweiz* (see section at the beginning of this chapter, Resources for the development of community-based palliative care). In the best case, the mandate comes from the relevant local government authority, the municipality. This ensures that the forum can be embedded sustainably within existing structures, that the local community are informed about the network, the network partners are able to position themselves more effectively, and that dying is recognized as a part of the life by the community.

Step 2: Constituting the core team

The core team is the driving force that enables a forum to be created. How the forum develops depends very much upon the composition of this group.
   The following aspects must therefore be taken into account:

a) The core team must reflect the different dimensions of palliative care and thus ensure the complete integration of all partners working in the palliative care sector. Depending on what is possible, the following key areas should be represented:
    •   General medical practice
    •   Outpatient care services
    •   Elderly and nursing homes
    •   Pastoral care
    •   Voluntary organizations/hospice services
    •   Political representatives/representatives of *palliative ostschweiz*.
b) Each representative additionally receives a mandate from their own sector to represent this sector in the core group. The experience of Eastern Switzerland shows that general practitioners have most difficulty with such integration and that the core group member who represents doctors must pay special attention to this issue.
c) The core group defines the main features of the forum and lays down the forum's approach, in consideration of existing regional conditions, the regulations of *palliative ostschweiz*, general guidelines of the municipality and the 'Community-based palliative care' handbook.
d) The group is usually led by the person who began the initiative and who set the first activities in motion. In general, this is also the person in charge of the flow of information between the forum and *palliative ostschweiz*, and who also takes part in platform discussions.

Experiences from the process

In each community, it is worthwhile considering who are the most important key actors, with the aim of persuading them to take part in the collaborative work. They are key contact persons and also those who recognize service gaps and weaknesses and are thus able to set a process of improvement and change in motion. The commitment of each of these key actors is needed if this process is to be successfully turned into action.

The affirmation of all general medical practitioners provided the AAR core group with a boost in terms of motivation. The support of doctors was thus a crucial factor, as without this professional group this project would have been seen by the core group members to have little purpose.

A survey at the palliative care centre in St. Gallen, which provides training courses for all doctors, shows that in the relevant municipalities not one general practitioner had yet received any basic training in palliative care.

Step 3: Integrating network partners

Every member of the core team provides a continual flow of information to organizations and institutions within their own sector about the development of the project. This encourages a sense of involvement in the forum itself.

The core team of the AAR forum decided at its first meeting to organize an event bringing together all the partners, to gather information on concerns, needs and questions, with the aim of identifying a clear mandate. The following organizations and institutions were invited to take part in this event:

- *Medical care*: general practitioners (GPs), consultants, e.g. psychiatrists, oncologists, etc.
- *Pastoral care*: churches, independent associations and representatives of other cultures and religions, e.g. Islam
- *Home sector*: all elderly and nursing homes in the catchment area
- *Outpatient care*: public and private Spitex providers (Spitex = out of hospital care/outpatient services), outpatient psychiatric care services and freelance care specialists in the region
- *Other sectors*: palliative bridging services (mobile palliative care service), St. Gallen outpatient hospice service, local authorities, physiotherapy, complementary medical services and *Pro Senectute* (an organization for the elderly)
- *Public authorities*

Depending on regional service provision, clinics and hospitals should also be involved as network partners.

Experiences from the process

Since this forum is partly hosted by the district authorities, which are to provide financial support where required, the three district authority leaders were kept personally informed and were approached to give their support.

Discussions with the three district authority leaders were surprisingly positive. All three confirmed their willingness to participate in the opening event and to provide general financial support. A central concern for all involved was that the inpatient sector, in this case the care/nursing homes, should be closely involved, and not only outpatient services.

Step 4: Awareness-raising

A *newspaper article* regarding the project's background, aims and planned implementation was published just before the launch event to raise public awareness. A freelance journalist was commissioned by the regional daily newspaper to write a report one week before the launch event about the plans to found the forum, its aims and background. The targeted involvement of media workers ensures that reportage can be reviewed before publication and that accurate information is thus provided to the wider public.

Launch event: the aims of this were to found the forum and define the mandate. The idea of a launch event was viewed as an effective way to bring together as many network partners as possible. At the event, following introductory greetings, the situation from the perspective of key sectors, outpatient care, home-based care, general practice and pastoral care was presented, together with the issues regarding community-based palliative care.

During the second part of the event, the intention was to enable space for a common conception regarding an active and productive network organization, which provides room for discussion, in order to reveal gaps in services, overlaps, misunderstandings and coordination and information needs. For this wider group, a suitable process method was required that would encourage constructive and creative exchange and the formulation of specific issues. For the Am Alten Rhein forum, we selected round-table discussions. These round tables were designed to include the widest possible mix of representatives from specialist professions to voluntary organizations with a moderator and an experienced specialist. Ideally, each round-table discussion comprised 7–9 individuals.

These round-table discussions brought to light a long list of ideas, concerns and tasks, which were then categorized within the wider group discussion according to the seven categories in Step 5 (see also table in Step 5) set out in the 'Community-based palliative care' handbook.

Experiences from the process

All participants in the launch event stated they were satisfied that they had been listened to and that their concerns had been taken up by the group. New relationships were formed, information was exchanged and coordination needs were discussed. The mandate for the core group was clearly defined and given out.

The constitution of the round-table discussions had to be carefully planned and directed, to facilitate the building of new connections wherever possible and the opportunity to learn from different perspectives. Care must however be taken not to allow too much leeway for potential latent competition, conflicts and social tensions between the individuals and organizations attending.

This form of exchange met with much positive approval. Feedback showed that participants felt able to contribute effectively, that discussion was well facilitated, and that when these issues were gathered together and listed, every contributor felt they had been accurately represented. Furthermore, the evaluation in the core group was felt to be clearly successful in addressing the questions, aspects, concerns and suggestions that had arisen.

Step 5: Implementing the results of the launch event

The concerns and questions of participants in the launch event were summarized and categorized as follows:

1 **Individuals/organizations**
   - What to do with uninformed doctors?
   - Goal: doctors to receive training in palliative care
   - Connecting doctors, Spitex, care professionals (homes)
   - Finding individuals within organizations
   - Specialization of homes (e.g. palliative care, dementia, etc.)
   - Who is the contact point, who is responsible, who connects different strands? ➔ clear structure
   - Pastoral care: individuals are not widely known
   - Worst case scenarios for homes/Spitex
   - Organization: no additional costs/no organizational superstructure
   - Using existing resources
   - No competitive approach (between homes, between doctors, etc.)
   - Social contact forms with/between non-Swiss individuals, e.g. Italians
2 **Coordinating care**
   - Reconsider medical regions
   - All those involved in a region have the same list (all involved palliative care organizations)

- Common schema and standards
- Palliative care treatment plan is desirable
- List: who is responsible in which sector, where and how are they accessible?
- Emergency structure (voluntary? professional?) for hospice services

3 **Voluntary sector input**
- Encouraging voluntary contributions, e.g. via training, showing appreciation
- Volunteer supervision
- Voluntary contributions from women's organizations, where are these?
- Seeking volunteers and providing training in various sectors (course costs)
- Volunteers require support
- Volunteer lists within villages, or brought in from outside?

4 **Round-the-clock continuity**
- No issues raised

5 **Communication**
- Forum – mutual exchange
- Addresses, knowledge about services
- Information brochure about services
- Communication about pastoral care
- Comparing experience
- Finding a common language
- Publicity and communications work

6 **An informed general public**
- Better information for the public regarding palliative care
- Better information for the public about regional service provision

7 **Controlling symptoms**
- Binding guidelines on standards
- Cultural differences (do the same standards always apply?)
- Harmonizing basic knowledge and training (homes, medical practitioners, Spitex, etc.)
- Developing standards (schema)
- Consistent schema for doctors

8 **Care for the dying**
- Improving conditions for those dying in homes
- Bridging service gaps (mobile palliative care services) for homes – funding?
- Place of death for young people: homes?
- Needs of terminally ill young people, services lacking, residential hospice?
- Funding palliative care for young people?

9 **Supporting relatives**
- Bereavement café, coordination with existing services?

- Cultural differences – other traditions
- Supporting relatives: peer support, ERFA (experience exchange) groups, etc.
- Hotline information (service provided by *palliative ostschweiz*)
- Establish network early on (e.g. organize funding aspects, etc.)

10 **Continuing learning**

- Palliative database, electronic?
- Palliative further training
- Literature/reading list for those requiring training
- IT pool, specialist expertise, further training

11 **Integration in the community and financial support**

Experiences from the process

The compilation of contributions made by participants was adopted as the mandate by the core group. Issues raised did not come as a surprise and confirmed the experiences of other forums.

This launch event also marked the official founding of the forum itself. As stipulated by regulations, an application for recognition as an official community-based forum was made to *palliative ostschweiz*.

Step 6: Defining priorities and planning

To establish an initial list of priorities for implementation, the core group defined foci based on the list given above and developed an implementation strategy. The following areas were identified for further development:

- Medicines information sheet
- Site-based documentation (basic information with addresses, staff list, procedure register)
- Professionals register and list of sources
- What to do in case of death (checklists to hand on)
- Voluntary services: steering group to be developed with interested parties.

Experiences from the process

The development of working groups to address specific issues meant that further individuals could be consulted, which promoted acceptance in the wider community and among the population. It was decided that all interested organizations, service providers and others with an interest in the issues should be kept informed of developments. They were to receive the list summarizing the contributions of those present at the launch event, together with a summary of priority measures for implementation.

Where the timing is right, the involvement of everyone concerned is effective, support is given by local authorities and a clear mandate exists, a small group working intensively together and showing great dedication can achieve a great deal within a short time in terms of setting up new regional networks and creating well-considered, pertinent and above all usable resources, which gain wide acceptance.

Step 7: Identifying the network partners, using the resources created by the core group

One year after the launch event, the selected materials are ready for use. The following three documents have been created:

• Palliative care treatment plan
• Checklist in case of death
• Comprehensive address list (institutions, authorities, palliative care services, medical practitioners, pastoral care providers, contact points for other cultures, etc.).

To ensure that these documents find acceptance and consistent application in palliative care situations, the network partners need to be effectively informed and provided with a guide to the background considerations to the documents.

The AAR forum is also organizing a further event, involving all those who took part in the launch event in information sessions and discussions.

Step 8: Public information and political leverage

The accompanying publicity activities through media involvement have on the one hand the aim of raising awareness among the general public about palliative care and on the other hand the goal of providing information to the public about what options are available in this respect within the region.

Experiences from the process

For the Am Alten Rhein forum, there appeared to be no need to define a single point of contact. The discussion made clear that each and every part of the network is also a point of contact and is able to provide impetus for whether and when the involvement of the network or a specific partner is required.

• The most important prerequisite is knowledge about the network and a clear decision about when to put this into practice.

The municipality should ideally provide a platform for publication of information via their homepage, and in any case should enable the printing of flyers. It is vital that the relevant authority (social services) should have access to such information.

Step 9: Longer-term planning of the forum

After setting up the forum itself, the focus should then lie with closing existing gaps in services and seeking solutions, but also with establishing the regular activities of a forum. This may include the following activities:

- Evaluating and adapting resource materials (e.g. palliative care treatment plan)
- Public relations activities
- Maintaining inter-professional cooperation at local level
- Regular information activities, meetings, further training provision through the network/forum
- Ensuring cooperation with *palliative ostschweiz* and other forums
- Undertaking activities in the context of International Hospice and Palliative Care Day.

Experiences from the process

The creation of a community-based care structure is not only of key importance for the palliative care sector. The developments in the health service in Switzerland (Bundesamt für Gesundheit – BAG, 2013) call for modern care structures that are conceived with a stronger emphasis upon the perspective of patients and less emphasis upon acute and inpatient care.

Integrated care pathways are already being implemented in various projects in Switzerland and are expected to find increasing application in the years ahead. Particularly where the establishment of a strategy on dementia is concerned (www.bag.admin.ch/themen/gesundheitspolitik/), as set out by the Federal Council, these structures are being increasingly demanded and also facilitated. Making use of existing community-based palliative care forums also in the framework of this strategy on dementia seems indispensable.

Community-based palliative care enables a dignified end of life

As a rule, basic ethical values that are more or less concretely formulated exist in organizations. Where an organization has set out such ethnical foundations in its mission statement, these normally function as explicitly desired and required values, to be observed by all those working in the organization. Yet implicit, that is not concretely defined, ethical values also characterize an organizational culture to a significant degree. A detailed analysis of the ethical values and their interplay as held by the various actors participating in local networks reveals the dimension of moral responsibility present in the implementation of this project. The following considerations clearly show that there are numerous implicit factors, which have an influence upon the development of palliative care in the community and which must be taken into account when setting up the forum.

Palliative care? Yes, we have been doing that for ages!

This sentiment is often expressed in the institutions and services providing care for critically ill and dying people. When we consider that most people wish to die at home, i.e. that the issue is about providing community-based care, then the burning question is: Could this statement and the attitude it reveals actually be hindering critically ill people from receiving 'true' palliative care services? Where specialist providers make such statements to the media and to politicians and decision makers, this can obstruct the real implementation of palliative care in practice. Indeed, it may even mean that critically ill people are prevented from receiving competent specialist palliative care!

People who have studied palliative care in detail often develop an inner passion either to become involved in the palliative care sector themselves, or to further develop their competence in this area, or to dedicate themselves to ensuring that this kind of care and treatment should be available for *all* people who need it. This inner passion is often fed by the fact that palliative care addresses and articulates the deepest of human needs. Of course one always thinks first of the physical aspects, which can be addressed in an objective and professional way and generally by means of scientifically proven treatments. Yet anyone who looks at palliative care at a deeper level cannot avoid encountering the fundamental ethical aspects of what it means to be human. These are basic values that we generally perceive as so self-evident that we never *explicitly* discuss them.

Palliative care, with its radical patient-focused approach, forces us to investigate, enquire about and recognize the fundamental values of the Other. This Other, suffering from an illness leading to their death, is in a dependent relationship with care professionals. In this context, communication among equals is important, as is providing the knowledge that will help the suffering person to make decisions about what their further care pathway might look like. The care professional should understand as much as possible about the person's history, experience and approach to life, so that comprehensible and appropriate services can be offered, the consequences and impacts of which are both understood and foreseen in terms of their significance and their effect.

Palliative care thus also implies a common way of looking at things, a common approach, and developing a concept, indeed a culture, that brings care specialists, sufferers and their relatives together. This is also at its heart about the question of what sort of culture is nurtured within organizations, and what importance is given to questions of preference and values, how autonomy is viewed, and whether the theme of the dignity of the terminally ill is actively addressed. Where an institution decides to explore these questions, the resources needed to do so are generally being made available. In an ideal case, a working group can take on the work of putting together and implementing a concept that addresses these issues. Following on from this, information, communication and public relations work are all supported and facilitated. In this sense, palliative care can also be seen as the 'tip of the iceberg' basis on an approach that sees the benefits of ethical guiding principles and inter-professional cooperation as self-evident.

> Where palliative care is seen as the tip of the iceberg, with a defined and practised approach based on mutual appreciation of values, respect and equality, the optimal conditions exist for other care and treatment concepts or for working with people who are suffering from chronic illness in a way that takes account of their dignity as individuals.

This shows that palliative care represents a comprehensive inter-professional care and treatment concept that at a fundamental level comprises a high degree of ethical awareness and patient-based approach, which should be understood by and be available to all, and at the same time, this should also enable those working in the sector to carry out professional or voluntary activities that enrich their understanding and their own sense of values.

This approach can and should be applied not only to the palliative care sector but should also be encouraged and nurtured in the community setting and in wider society. Palliative care after all sees itself not as a culture of single institutions. Although single institutions can help those requiring such care to have some of their needs met, a care handover is often also required, for example when the outpatient setting reaches its limits, when a nursing home or palliative care ward can provide a level of service that is seen as more appropriate to the situation, even temporarily, as a transition or short-term intervention in order to stabilize the situation at home once again.

Dignity in dependency

When people become ill, old and/or require care, they become to some extent dependent upon organizations. Sometimes, there is a choice as to which organization or residential arrangement can be considered. Often, however, it is less a question of choice than of necessity. In this context, a person requiring care enters into a state of dependency – and it is at this point that the responsibility of organizations begins.

Where I am understood, I am also listened to, acknowledged and accepted, I am valued and respected as a human being. This means that when in my dependent relationship my own needs are included and solutions are sought,

I feel that I am understood, respected and at home. This sense of dignity is put at risk when a person is suddenly no longer recognized as a subject and a tendency develops for them to be treated as an object and the issue becomes one of 'maintenance' or 'management' of the person (von Schirach, 2014).

The culture in organizations

A specific culture within an institution is not simply a given. In general, it grows with the people who live within it. It is important that the strategic level recognizes that an organizational culture nurtured in a conscious way is necessary, and that this requires the explicit investment of time and attention. A culture such as this must be actively implemented, maintained, encouraged and evaluated. It is only in this way that impact and sustainability can be created and a new culture of living can emerge as a result.

This culture of living is particularly indispensable where critically ill and dying people are concerned, and it forms the basis of palliative care. This means that it is not a culture of dying that must be created but rather a culture of living, which also places quality of life at the heart of the experience of dying.

The culture of living and quality of life does not represent a service that can be calculated or paid for, but rather a philosophical approach, which must be nurtured within an organization. Palliative care is often understood merely as concepts and options for relieving suffering and facilitating death. Thus according to a person's level of knowledge, this philosophical approach is either completely ignored or is entirely taken for granted, i.e. implicitly included, when palliative care is discussed. If the principles of palliative care are to be brought to life in a sustainable and effective way, the foundations, the ethical considerations, must either already be in place or they must be addressed during the implementation process.

The forum as a space for reflection and ethical exploration

The community-based network from which the forums emerge faces the particular challenge of respecting the autonomy and culture of the individual organizations and institutions, while finding a pathway through mutual exchange towards a nuanced approach and culture that is capable of building a common basis for all the network partners. The forum sees itself therefore as a networking platform between institutions, organizations and voluntary organizations and political authorities in the region. The focus of the forum lies with debating the different outlooks of the individual institutions and organizations and finding consensus, with the aim of applying precisely these fundamental ethical principles to the care, treatment and support they provide to people in palliative situations. This requires that these principles are taken into account both in the constitution and in the design of collaborative work within the new organization, i.e. the forum.

On one hand, the members of the core group must be carefully selected, since they must represent their area of specialism, their service or their organization. On the other hand, they must also be able to bring questions, information and concerns back to the forum, and in every case be able to address and discuss these.

The four founding principles (Bürgi, 2009) are the prerequisite for authentic, personally coherent decision-making. They can be formulated in concrete terms in these four questions: Can I be a member of this organization? Do I want to be a member of this organization? Can I be myself here? What are the benefits of what I do here? In this way, the personal involvement of individuals plays a crucial role in the development of well-functioning and lively forums.

Reflecting upon economic principles in the forum

Other themes, such as demographic change, austerity politics and changes caused by the introduction of diagnosis related groups (DRGs) in Swiss hospitals, have also created other needs and other medical and care requirements where primary care institutions at municipal level are concerned. Institutions and organizations are increasingly becoming aware that they cannot or do not need to fulfil all service provision by themselves, or that this simply cannot be funded through their regular sources.

Local networks within the community can create a counterweight, which provides space on the one hand for the needs of sufferers to be focused upon and on the other for the professionals and volunteers in the sector to exchange experience and thoughts, to reflect upon the issues at hand or just to gain a breathing space and recharge their batteries in the company of others with experience of similar situations. Economizing in a positive sense has a role to play here, too, through the aspect of good provision, where economic considerations can ensure continuity in the operation of specialist and pastoral care (Manzeschke, 2010).

What positive changes can forums create?

Macro level

Society recognizes that when someone is terminally ill and death is approaching, a network should be available. It is understood that trusted individuals, whom one may have known over many years through a number of crises, have a part to play and that when these trusted individuals no longer know what to do, other network partners will come forward and provide further help.

This understanding can also aid considerations regarding assisted suicide or may prevent or alleviate the development of depression and anxiety. Quality of life is not an empty turn of phrase, but rather has a renewed and important role to play precisely in situations of health crisis and at the end of life.

Meso level

Professional groups that generally operate with a high degree of independence and initiative recognize the value of joint development of constructive communication, cooperation and coordination. Those who work alone also find support in the common aim that being able to lead a life with dignity and to end one's life with the same dignity should be the right of all people. Putting inter-professionalism into practice cannot be experienced as a loss of specific identification and independence but rather as gaining specialist knowledge, expanded perspectives, the fulfilment of the patient-based approach, needs-based services and, under certain circumstances, also gaining resilience among professionals.

Micro level

The network is brought together first and foremost for the individual sufferers and their families. It does not serve a collective purpose but should rather answer individual needs and provide the necessary framework to allow self-determination and autonomy to flourish. Yet the professionals and volunteers also find a 'home' in their work. Different professional groups work on the basis of equality with one another, which gives individual workers a sense of mutual respect and of belonging; in other words, it creates quality of life within daily work too.

The challenges so far

It was clear from the beginning that doctors had to be convinced by the idea of the forum. It was a key concern of the core team member who represented medical practitioners that all their colleagues should support this work and be well informed about each step along the way. This was not successful to the same extent in every case.

Connecting the service providers engaged in the same or similar work within a network may be seen as representing a particular challenge, for example in the case of public and private providers of outpatient care services. In the Am Alten Rhein region, this was happily not the case. A sense of collegiate cooperation had existed before, characterized by the understanding that 'in care and treatment, all kinds and different kinds of services are needed'. Thus, for example, the webpage www.info-alter-nativen.ch offers the opportunity to publish their details to a range of different local providers of inpatient and outpatient care and advice services.

Raising awareness among the general public is a constant theme during the set-up phase of the forums, and in future it is clear that more attention must be paid to this aspect. It is increasingly observed that voluntary organizations such as mother and women's associations, and often also those voluntary organizations hosted by the churches, are either in sharp decline or have ceased to exist altogether. This is a challenge that can only be partly addressed in the context of setting up a forum.

The immediate future of the forums

In the immediate future, the forums will have to deal with extremely pragmatic issues: whether in future a defined point of contact with a telephone helpline might be developed by the forum is something that will have to be clarified on a regional basis. In Switzerland, so-called hotlines dealing with all questions surrounding palliative care are being developed for both sufferers and professionals. At the moment, these are primarily available on a regional basis, but it may also be the case that a supra-regional or national helpline will be developed. It seems important that either telephone calls should be sent through directly to the relevant region or that knowledge about regional networks and hotlines should be easily available.

How much structure in supra-organization needs to be provided is the subject of lively discussion within *palliative ostschweiz*. Initially, a flyer template is to be developed, with the minimal but necessary information, which can be added to by individual forums and either made available via the homepages of local municipalities or in printed form for the general public.

The founding documents created by forums, such as standards, palliative care plans or checklists should be made available for others to use as a resource. Duplicated efforts and overlaps should be avoided, so that materials and resources can be used efficiently and above all effectively in the service of sufferers.

Lessons learned

The founding of the forums should strengthen community-based palliative care in Eastern Switzerland. The clear wish expressed by Swiss men and women to be able to die at home should be fulfilled for a greater number of people through the work of the forums.

While the forums are being set up, common basic principles will be developed and network partners learn to identify with these principles and with the local network. They see themselves as a part of a greater whole, which functions at local level and offers a point of contact for sufferers and their families within the local community. Every contact point operates in the knowledge that it has the backing of the local network and can activate this at any time.

Central to the idea of 'compassionate communities' is the key concept that it should be possible to bring death and dying (back again) into the community and to open up opportunities for local people to determine how their own final phase of life will be (cf. Kellehear, 2005). The forums are anchored in the local community, they see the municipalities as their partners and they enable negotiations over basic principles in the very locations in which these basic principles are intended to ensure that life is lived to the very end in dignity. We view the forums as an important step in the direction of greater compassion in our communities in Eastern Switzerland.

Notes

1   The area includes the cantons of Appenzell Ausserrhoden, Appenzell Innerrhoden, Glarus, St. Gallen, Thurgau and the Principality of Liechtenstein.
2   Forum documents/regulations. www.palliative-ostschweiz.ch

References

Bundesamt für Gesundheit – BAG (2013) *Die gesundheitspolitischen Prioritäten des Bundesrates. Gesundheit 2020. Eidgenössisches Departement des Innern (EDI).* Bern.
Bundesamt für Statistik – BFS (2009) *Statistiken der stationären Gesundheitsversorgung – Studie zu den letzten Lebensjahren im Heim und Spital.* Bern.
Bürgi, D. (2009) Pflegende unterstützen. *Zeitschrift der Gesellschaft für Logotherapie und Existenzanalyse* 1: 35–39.
Eychmüller, S. and Domeisen, B.F. (2013) Community palliative care in Switzerland: from assessment to action. In: Hockley, J., Froggatt, K. and Heimerl, K. (eds) *Participatory Research in Palliative Care. From Action to Reflection.* Oxford: Oxford University Press, 75–85.
GfK Switzerland AG (2010) *Repräsentative Bevölkerungsbefragung Palliative Care, im Auftrag des Bundesamt für Gesundheit (BAG).* Kellehear, A. (2005) *Compassionate Cities. Public Health and End-of-Life Care.* London: Routledge.
Kumar, S. (2007) Kerala, India: a regional community-based palliative care model. *Journal of Pain and Symptom Management,* 33: 623–627.
Manzeschke, A. (2010) Spiritualität und Ökonomie – Fundamentalethische Überlegung zu ihrer diakonischen Verhältnisabstimmung. In: Schoenauer, H. (ed.) *Spiritualität und innovative Unternehmensführung.* Stuttgart: Kohlhammer, 2011, 566–574.
Palliativzentrum Kantonsspital St. Gallen (undated) *Palliative Care in der Gemeinde. Ein Handbuch zur Vernetzung. Erfahrungen aus einer Ostschweizer Studie.* St. Gallen.
Saunders, C. (1984) The philosophy of terminal care. In: Saunders, Cicely (ed.) *The Management of Terminal Malignant Disease,* 2nd edition. London: Edward Arnold, 232–241 (1st edition in 1978).
von Schirach, F. (2014) *Die Würde ist antastbar.* München: Piper.

13 Dementia-friendly communities

Together for a better life with (and without) dementia

Reimer Gronemeyer and Verena Rothe

Initiator: *Aktion Demenz*

The non-profit association *Aktion Demenz* is a German-wide initiative that developed out of the 2006 workshop 'Together for a Better Life with Dementia', organised by the Robert Bosch Foundation (Robert Bosch Stiftung, 2007). It aims to improve the lives of people with (and without) dementia, primarily through public dialogue, and to raise awareness for this variation or manifestation of life. Trying to counteract the medicalisation of dementia by 'resocialising' it, *Aktion Demenz* aims to reduce stigmatisation and bring about social change. It includes people from all areas of society, who are committed to working towards more tolerance for and better inclusion of people with dementia and their families and friends via local projects.

In 2007, *Aktion Demenz* initiated a public discourse on how citizens affected by dementia could be approached openly and in a spirit of solidarity within local communities. The various efforts and projects that responded to this call and attempted to put its aims into practice were presented in autumn 2008 as part of a two-day event entitled '*Aufbruch*' ('new beginning') (Kreutzner and Rothe, 2009). The event ended with the reading of a statement calling for a better life for those with dementia ('*Esslinger Aufruf für ein besseres Leben mit Demenz*'; *Aktion Demenz*, 2008), which was then signed by participants and has been further publicised ever since.

In partnership between *Aktion Demenz* and the Robert Bosch Foundation, the idea arose to create a funding programme to support local efforts aligned with our common goals. Funded by the Robert Bosch Foundation, *Aktion Demenz* initiated the 2008 funding programme 'People in the Community Living with Dementia', which has been implemented three times since then. This provided funding to local projects with a focus on dementia that initiate as well as implement community-based activities aimed at supporting people with dementia and enabling their participation in society: 78 selected local initiatives were given not only moral but also financial support. These projects are also presented online at *www.demenzfreundliche-kommunen. de* (at the time of writing, available in German only).

This programme was characterised by its active consideration of and support for smaller initiatives that are otherwise often hindered by formal application processes. All applications were considered in detail to ensure that not only professional fundraisers and experienced project leaders were taken into account. This has proven to be especially valuable in relation to supporting grassroots projects and the efforts of individuals.

However, it became clear that a formal application process still discourages and deters such initiatives. In some cases, these are unable to provide a legal entity that could apply for funding to begin with. Additionally, programmes such as this are primarily shared and promoted within the domain they are most commonly associated with – in this case, health and social care. Although there is increasing awareness of the relevance of dementia in domains other than health and social care, even in the third iteration of the programme, the call was not always forwarded to institutions in other sectors, such as culture, family, youth, leisure or migration, or distributed among faith groups, clubs, societies and schools.

However, despite these hurdles, we were successful in taking our approach to the supported communities and the general public, and even inspired Europe-wide initiatives (for example the programme 'Living Well with Dementia in the Community', www.nef-europe.org/efid). After the first year (with 150 applications, 13 projects) had served as a test run for putting the idea of a *dementia-friendly community* into practice, the second iteration (234 applications, 37 projects) was already far more comprehensive and diverse, both geographically (within Germany) as well as in terms of topics and breadth of focus. The focus of the third and last iteration of the programme (155 applications, 28 projects) was on developing individual aspects of the approach of dementia-friendly communities in more detail and improving its transfer to other domains. This is the reason why insights gained in recent years will be published separately.[1]

Societal background

Seeing challenge as chance

The current age distribution in our society is unmatched in history. Simultaneously, social structures that could support people confronted with dementia are diminishing. People are slowly becoming aware of the fact that the number of people suffering from dementia is increasing and will continue to do so. They are beginning to understand that dementia is a growing social, cultural, economic and humanitarian challenge for German society. Despite this, they have not yet been sufficiently sensitised to the situation. There is a lack of new concepts that take into account individuals, families, communities and society at large. Currently, the focus is placed only on dementia itself and on individuals with dementia. However, it also needs to be directed at society and social development. It is an important function of society to support individuals living with dementia, to value their resources and abilities, and to involve them in everyday life. Dementia must not be pushed into a medical-pharmacological ghetto to avoid having to deal with the social and cultural needs that it creates.

Without question, dementia is a consequence of a rapidly ageing society. It is safe to assume that dementia

- and its increasing prevalence trigger fears,
- encourages technocratic solutions,
- runs the risk of being only poorly managed due to limited funds,
- overburdens traditional health and social care institutions,
- exhausts family and friends,
- and will overwhelm the healthcare budget,

which will have unforeseeable consequences both for those directly concerned and society at large.

The spread of dementia is bound to lead to crises in all areas of social life, on an individual as well as a general level. For example, if nothing is done, one day, deteriorating care conditions of people with dementia could be presented as acceptable in the media (through the use of descriptive labels, such as 'useless eaters', etc.).

At *Aktion Demenz*, we propose that dementia be seen not as a threat but as a chance to invest in our care system and encourage volunteer work and to rethink and reform structures of family, friendship and community to make them more dementia-friendly. We believe that a society that treats people with dementia well is almost automatically taking the right steps towards becoming a society that values life. Dementia shakes our personality and self-image to the core. We need to tackle the questions that dementia raises and to see people with dementia as 'messengers' who call on us to revolutionise an environment that is becoming more and more hostile to life. The urgency of this message is not only visible in 'number games' and statistical projections, but also in the actual realities of life. These realities have changed drastically in recent years and will continue to do so.

A tendency towards social isolation has developed, because there are fewer marriages and more divorces than previously, together with a decreasing average number of children in families, and the growing distances between the households of parents and their children, due to the demand for mobility and flexibility (Peuckert, 2012). However, social networks have positive effects on psychological health and competence in old age and can even prevent or alleviate symptoms of Alzheimer's. Most importantly, they play a vital role in enabling people to age with dignity without becoming isolated and lonely. Unfortunately, due to the growing number of people affected, the decline of familial support networks, and economic limitations in the health and social care sectors, people with dementia are at risk of becoming excluded culturally and socially as well as no longer being treated with dignity. In the future, there will be fewer and fewer family members in the classical sense available for care, and eventually also an ongoing decline in the numbers of financial supporters, professional care workers, etc.

Diagnosing a dementia-hostile world

We are currently creating a world 'with which we are unable to keep pace, and which surpasses the capacities of both our emotions and our responsibility whenever we try to comprehend it', as Günther Anders (1980: 18; our translation) already expressed this concern in the middle of the twentieth century.

Since then, society has become overtly hostile towards dementia. We wish to argue that it is not people with dementia who distance themselves from others, but that society has distanced itself so far from those who have lost their way that they simply cannot find their way back again. This seems especially obvious when looking at the following circumstances that frame the position of dementia in our societies.

The crisis of communality

Our industrial society of constant growth has turned us into isolated consumers. But we are more than that, which is why we need to break out of this prison of automatisation. No longer being part of a larger community is one of modernity's most daunting phenomena. Living in communities, however, is founded on smaller scales and locally organised structures, networks and groups of friends. That is what we need, even if our world view is still based on fragmentation and isolation (Shiva, 2009: 269, our translation).

Zygmunt Baumann (2007) provides an acute analysis of this crisis of communality, which particularly affects people with dementia, and discusses the ongoing dissolution of social bonds and social cohesion through modernisation:

> To the acclaim of some enthusiastic observers of the new trends, the void left behind by citizens massively retreating from the extant political battlefields to be reincarnated as consumers is filled by ostentatiously non-partisan and ruggedly unpolitical 'consumer activism'.
> (Baumann, 2007: 146)

Our ageing society is faced with exponentially increasing problems, such as the financing of pensions, rising demands to the healthcare system and increasing healthcare costs, growing demand for care, and the social isolation of the elderly (Siegrist, 2010: 89).

The crisis of community

In our current system, money and (decision-making) power seems to become more and more centralised while social issues are pushed back into communities' spheres of responsibility. Power is globalised, while social catastrophes are localised. Dementia, a future social hot spot, has increasingly come into focus since the 1980s. While it was initially approached from a medical perspective only, it has become clear that this does not go far enough. Making dementia a community issue must not mean simply outsourcing it as a problem for communities to dispose of.

The crisis of the individual

Members of our society are becoming increasingly unable to meet the demands of the culture of urgency to which they are exposed (cf. Bindé, 2010). Depression has become an epidemic, burnout is widespread and psychopathologies are on the increase. Modern individuals have clearly reached their limits and dementia only adds to this phenomenon. Anders (1980: 16) describes what he calls the 'Promethean gap', with people lounging around between their various appliances like bewildered dinosaurs. People with dementia are illustrative examples of this. In a symbolic yet challenging way, they question the self-conception of modernity as the refusal to owe anything to anyone. Promethean pride refers to the idea of owing everything, including one's self, only to oneself (Anders, 1980: 24). One of the drastic examples of this was the suicide of Gunter Sachs, the German multimillionaire and industrialist, who related his decision to end his life to his fear that he might have Alzheimer's, despite having no such diagnosis.

The shame that people with dementia feel is an expression of this trait of modern societies and exposes its inadequacy and coldness. Our society – obsessed with consumption and competition – sees people with dementia as failures because of their slowness, their inability to be 'productive members of society', etc.

It is therefore not enough that communities take on a few select 'measures' to improve the care for people with dementia. Dementia forces us to think about a new beginning in terms of the social relationships between modern citizens. In a disquieting way, it turns the strengths of modern society into weaknesses: billion-bit memory storage becomes memory loss, excessive individualisation turns into loss of personality. Dementia is the return of the tenets of modernity – flexibility! acceleration! autonomy! – as caricatures. It challenges us, in a way that is both frightening and liberating, to rebuild our societies from the ground up. How do we want to treat people who are seen by some as 'no longer useful', who cost money, who can no longer compete, who might even be unable to consume? Do we want to shunt them out of the way, have them cared for or even 'dispose' of them? Or do we want to see them as an opportunity for seeking out and imagining new ways, a new sociality, a new culture of helping?

According to a quote often attributed to Mahatma Gandhi, 'we need to be the change we wish to see in the world' – this is no less true for dementia and how we approach it.

Paving the way to dementia-friendly communities

The concept of dementia-friendly communities

The social context discussed above is the reason for the call by *Aktion Demenz* for dementia-friendly communities, i.e. communities in which people with dementia and their families can live comfortably and are included not only in theory but in their lived realities. Community is used here to refer to various levels: municipal communities, towns, cities, districts, neighbourhoods and small-scale communities.

Without relieving political actors of their responsibility in this matter, we want to stress that the social, political, economic and humanitarian challenges we face can only be tackled if forms of shared responsibility are developed and put into practice both by cities and towns and on the communal level. It is in the community where citizens, politicians and other local actors can identify networks of contacts and support as well as create new ones. They have to partially reinvent their communities to effect actual positive change for people with dementia. Both shared reflection and direct local action are prerequisites for building a dementia-friendly community.

It is a common but false belief that the crucial point of such change lies in more and better care and consultation services, volunteer care work, raising awareness for dementia on the level of communal administration or networking individual actors within the care infrastructure with the aim of making the latter more efficient. All these are undoubtedly important steps towards a society that is more amenable to both people with dementia and those who attend to them. However, *Aktion Demenz* wants to look – and go – further and pursue a more far-reaching vision with its call for dementia-friendly communities.

To put it bluntly, we need to develop a more friendly attitude towards dementia. Living with dementia is anything but easy and often means a great deal of suffering for those involved. However, how we see dementia and how we treat those who live with dementia both have a profound impact on how dementia affects those living with it and how it develops. A better life with dementia starts in our minds.

We hope to create dementia-friendly communities through supportive structures, awareness-raising, specific projects and events, opportunities for people with and without dementia to meet one another, creating connections between all generations and professions, help among neighbours, and citizen activism.

Some efforts such as these have already been identified and additional local initiatives have been encouraged (cf. Gronemeyer et al., 2007), from projects on the interactions between dementia and migration/art/youth to campaigns for awareness-raising, networking, etc.

The many ways in which people with dementia can be socially included that also contribute to a change in social awareness include joint guided tours in museums for people with and without dementia; 'dementia companions' in clubs, societies and faith groups; joint sports activities; trainings for e.g. fire service staff and people working in retail or in administration on how to treat people with dementia; everyday ordinary interactions with people with dementia; and casual help in everyday situations.

In Walldorf in Baden-Württemberg, people with and without dementia, young and old, on foot or in wheelchairs, with prams or walking frames, are coming together to take a walk and talk to one another. In Minden-Lübbecke in North Rhine-Westphalia, a project organised by the initiative 'living with dementia', local sports clubs and the German Cyclists' Association offers joint bicycle tours for people with and without dementia, as well as other activities. In Cologne, an initiative is trying to enable cultural participation for people who are being cared for in homes as museum educators are trying to open up to this new audience. Also in Cologne, two church communities are becoming dementia-friendly, which means that members of the church who show signs of dementia can continue to sing in the church choir, visit the church café and attend mass. In Wiesbaden in Hesse, an artist is trying to explore the artistic potential of people with dementia with his project '*Blickwechsel*' ('change of perspective'). Finally, in Munich, people with and without dementia are working together to create a shared meeting space.

One important aspect of these initiatives is the effort to try to bring people with and without dementia together in their local communities. This can lead to better mutual understanding and lasting improvements in the lives of people with dementia and their family and friends. An open, sympathetic environment can alleviate the development of dementia as well as its effects, directly and indirectly, and have a positive influence on the community in general. This is one reason why we hope – and we are happy to report that this is happening already – that the funded projects will inspire other communities to develop their own ideas and projects, benefiting from the experience of others.

The ideas and demands of dementia-friendly communities – a new culture of mutual support – are clearly applicable to other domains of life as well, such as the ways in which we deal with and treat

- age in general,
- our own as well as others' mortality,
- other groups that are marginalised and/or need special care,
- ways of interacting more generally.

What could a dementia-friendly community look like?

No organisation or individual should be allowed to define with authority how dementia-friendly communities should operate and how they should be implemented. Instead, suggestions for possible models arise from conversations between all local actors, including those directly affected by dementia. This, however, requires a shared understanding of the challenges we face, and a new way of 'doing community'. This is the reason why, strictly speaking, there are no dementia-friendly communities yet, but rather communities on their way to becoming dementia-friendly.

The most important goal is shaping the community as a social space in such a way that people with dementia and their families and friends can lead pleasant – 'ordinary' – lives. For this, they need to be able to participate. Participation is a human right and obligates communities to make life within the community, its infrastructure and other services inclusive and accessible. However, this will not suffice by itself to create a new culture of mutual support, to rethink communities and to live accessibility in our minds. We need to change how dementia and people with dementia are perceived, we need to end their stigmatisation and we need to initiate lasting changes in awareness. Similar to how we have already begun to make our streets and houses physically accessible, we now need to make and keep communities and society free of barriers for people with dementia and other impairments.

Whether they are dealing with less pronounced forms of disorientation or with dementia in its late stages, people with dementia need not only high-quality medical care and nursing but also social interaction with others, an understanding environment, the feeling of (still) being a part of their neighbourhoods, towns and communities. They also need the sympathy of others, not as paternalistic aid but as honest care – and caring – that is seen as a normal facet of everyday life. This, too, requires new and different ways of treating each other and offering casual mutual support (cf. Kreutzner and Rothe, 2009).

Creating dementia-friendly communities means creating humane communities that are friendly environments for everyone in them. This requires larger-scale social transformation and more solidarity between individuals. Inclusion and participation require us all to be ready to tear down old, inaccessible structures and transform current ones. Every one of us needs to face this topic and any potential fears related to it in their private as well as public lives, to practise encountering people with dementia as an unexceptional facet of everyday life, and to accept the changes that come with this.

The following points could be of importance for concrete local efforts when trying to effect such a change in awareness and allow people with dementia to live a life of social inclusion:

- creating and raising public awareness,
- encouraging encounters between people with and without dementia,

- developing ideas and models of shared responsibility and cooperation that involve all local actors and citizens,
- adapting local circumstances to local needs (e.g. accessibility, infrastructure, help among neighbours),
- exploring creative approaches to dementia in art and culture.

If local administrations as well as political actors realised that dementia, before anything else, is prompting us to imagine social solutions and new social networks, they could offer valuable contributions to supporting civil society initiatives and create an environment in which communities can deal with the topic of dementia, de-stigmatise it and foster the inclusion of people with dementia (see for example Stadt Arnsberg, 2011). For example, they can analyse existing structures to find deficits in their own communities. They can find, initiate and develop local forms of support, and connect local actors by initiating round-table discussions and working groups, or take part in and support already existing ones. They can function as a neutral partner and moderate the planning of projects as well as engage in cooperatively conducted projects for and with people with dementia. In particular, they can promote non-work-based systems of help and support as well as connect them to professional efforts. At the same time, individual steps and diverse smaller and independent initiatives coming from all domains of social life remain crucially important.

Even though this is often neglected, dementia also affects children and teenagers, for example as grandchildren of people with dementia, as children of friends and family who care for people with dementia, or as carers themselves. They are also part of a generation that will have to find ways of meeting the rising number of people with dementia with dignity and in a supportive fashion and will probably have to create stable social networks more independently than the generations before them (cf. Philipp-Metzen, 2008).

Aktion Demenz does not wish to give a final answer to the question of what dementia-friendly communities look like or how the goal of implementing such communities can be reached. What is important is channelling discussions, suggestions, examples, ideas, campaigns and experiences into local projects and ideas, and showing that communities that work to face the challenges of dementia work to achieve a better future for all (cf. Gronemeyer and Wißmann, 2008).

Selection of experiences from the funding programme 'People in the Community Living with Dementia'

We will now discuss some aspects of a qualitative evaluation of the second and third iterations of the project, led by Charlotte Jurk, which we are going to supplement with our experiences with the 78 projects that have been funded by the programme in Germany so far.

- The projects met the intended range, variety and difference in terms of starting context and implementation.
- Many families, especially in rural areas, expect that they should be able to deal with the 'problem' themselves without any external help.
- In many cases, the people involved in the projects have different expectations of how these are to be implemented. While professionals may say, 'We need to put together a brochure', family and friends might think, 'Why a brochure? All we need is a piece of paper.'
- Projects targeting smaller-scale social spaces are seen as more successful than those that target overly large areas. If outreach work is spread too thinly, this often leads to uncertainty as to whether or how the project's goals have been achieved. In comparison, changes in more concentrated and familiar local areas are felt more easily.
- The greater the extent to which a project has been built on volunteer actions, the more directly it has reached those affected by dementia and their family and friends.
- The already strongly visible trend for boundaries between volunteering and semi-professionalism to become increasingly permeable (which sometimes also affects family and friends) needs to be critically evaluated:

> The more weight is put on certificates and trainings and the more volunteer work is 'upgraded' into a (badly) paid service, the greater the danger that instead of offering simple and practical support to those who need it, all that is happening is the creation of new market demands (a professional carer for every person with dementia). This way, rather than developing a new culture of community, volunteer work is bound into an exclusionary demand for expert professionalism. To make the situation worse, many volunteers actually already rely on their work to secure their livelihoods.
>
> (Jurk, 2012: S. 39; our translation)

- To effect change in everyday life, public as well as individual awareness must be fine-tuned to notice seemingly small changes which only slowly accumulate into social interaction, need time and patience, and are often overlooked – but can lead to significant changes over longer periods of time.
- Generally, communities seem to be quick to pass on the topic of dementia to charity organisations and volunteers. In particular, financial support and long-term commitment remain rare (cf. Jurk, 2012).

Additionally, it is important to stress that dementia is a cross-cutting issue that should not be treated in isolation but that should be considered when dealing with other issues as well.

Two areas where visible change has taken place in recent years are retail and administration. While at first attitudes such as 'People with dementia? We don't have those here' or even 'We don't believe in social activism' were common, now that the market value of the elderly – and thereby of those living with dementia – has increased, it seems as if trainings on dementia are being conducted every other day (often by volunteers who do not get paid for these) and are then advertised by businesses in an attempt to attract customers. However, the skills being taught in such trainings are often not about dementia-friendly communities but about market-oriented aspects, such as supporting care and distribution systems and 'tracking down' people with dementia.

One major difficulty in understanding the idea of dementia-friendly communities lies in its underlying change of perspective. There is a difference between, on the one hand, building networks of fire service staff, hospital workers, bus drivers, retail workers, members of clubs and societies, administrators, professionals and the general population with the aim of catching 'demented' people when they 'escape' from their supervision to prevent something – in the worst case, something life-threatening – happening to them and, on the other hand, building a community to support people with dementia so they can participate in everyday life with or without others' assistance for as long as possible and do not need to retreat due to shame or other forms of resistance as quickly as they do now.

While sensitising and training certainly have positive aspects, it is important to keep in mind that knowledge is always relative. Particularly in relation to Alzheimer's disease, many questions – both about the phenomenon itself and about affected individuals – are still unanswered and can often not simply be answered by a yes or a no.

As some businesses and organisations have shown, effective measures for compensating for age-related difficulties can also be implemented without any special training. For example, some banks offer reading glasses for their elderly and visually impaired customers to help them fill out forms. The organisers of a carnival parade compensated for the disorientation of one of their members by assigning him to a position in the safer centre of the train. On the one hand, this shows that people with no special training can and do come up with supportive and practical ideas. On the other hand, it reminds us that there is still a lot left to imagine, develop and try differently.

In our modern age – an age that is marked by the importance of measurable results, numbers and facts – it is more important than ever that we see social issues as processes, take the time we need and try to include others for the long term. Only then will we be able to involve people from areas of life other than our own and prevent organisational blindness through inspiration from the outside. Unfortunately, it is still only rarely recognised how important it is to not only tolerate or try to commission civil activism and engagement, but to actively pursue, support and allow it to develop on its own.

In a world that has become highly specialised – and this applies to both society at large and the 'dementia scene' – it is crucial to perform activities as a community, to simply come together, not asking *who* is coming but *why* they are coming. With all the many niche offers for people with dementia, one might start to think they will all develop into a 'dementia town' such as the one in the Netherlands (see www.vivium.nl/hogewey). Such things may be efficient, but they are also artificial. Those involved will find positive aspects, but mostly in the form of 10-minute activation. Such offers could perhaps form a tiny part of a dementia-friendly community but they by no means fully encompass our vision of such a community. Where is the life in them, where is the everyday, the things that do not work right away, the challenges that sometimes also allow for growth and evolving, where is the spontaneity, where are incidental meetings, exchanges and learning from all kinds of different people? It is concerning that these offers are taken up so quickly because they are seen as a simple and fast 'solution'. If we want to create inclusive and dementia-friendly communities, dementia must be understood as a cross-cutting issue that is not cut off from all others. We need to focus on community, on integration and on acceptance of all those who are easily marginalised, not just people with dementia.

Against this background, possibilities and moments of shared experience and community between people with and without dementia are all the more positive. People who dare to dip their toes into such encounters most often find their expectations surpassed. We should keep this in mind in an environment where working with dementia is sometimes based on the idea that unrehearsed encounters should be avoided. The fact that attendants at dementia-related events often ask how they should react when they meet someone with dementia is proof that the current trend towards professionalisation also produces ever-greater insecurities. It is all the more liberating when these people then experience new situations in a more positive way, without their fears and insecurities blocking an exchange.

The question of how one should react is often answered by listing the usual strategies: showing appreciation, being respectful, trying to enter and understand the other's own personal world, etc. However, we also have to ask an even bigger question: How, in our increasingly sectionalised and specialised world, can we meet others, those foreign to us, in the first place? How can we meet others who are 60 or even 70 years younger, coming from a different country or culture? These encounters are not easy, but they are possible, and they are an adventure that is more easily embarked upon if we trust the moment as well as our human senses and empathy rather than merely relying on professional support. One might say that not much can happen in these encounters without professional mediation – yet surely, all the small yet crucial facets of everyday human interaction do.

What happens when we rely on the idea that nothing can go wrong if we only learn how to behave 'properly'? How does this affect our actual interactions with people? Which other approaches and how much direct and immediate contact does this prevent? It is not our aim to downplay the consequences of dementia, but it is important and, ultimately, rewarding to think about 'otherness' in a more general sense, and about how it frequently leads to exclusion.

The success of the concept of dementia-friendly communities and why we should also be somewhat sceptical of it

As discussed above, *Aktion Demenz* has focused on the idea of dementia-friendly communities in recent years. This idea has been met with much positive feedback and, thanks to the funding by the Robert Bosch Foundation, has made dementia a topic of discussion in many communities. While dementia is still an issue dominated by medicine and medical institutions, public discourse is slowly shifting towards recognising its social sides as well. *Aktion Demenz* has focused on this social aspect and has, along with other actors, contributed to furthering this aspect of the discussion. A social model of dementia and its relation to communities has been taken up outside Germany, too. *Aktion Demenz* will continue to work to open up the medical monoculture in which approaches to dementia are still embedded and to make dementia a focus for civil society. The framework in which this work is conducted requires more sustained, ongoing reflection and discussion.

The success of the concept of dementia-friendly communities brings with it many possibilities but also some dangers. It is easily misunderstood, which is why we feel the need to stress once again that we do not see dementia-friendly communities as yet another building block in the expansion of the institutionalised care system in which communal structures are simply another service layer between care homes and families. Nor do we intend them as a rather sly and subtle strategy for relieving the welfare state by outsourcing care services that are no longer affordable to the cost-effective substructures of volunteer work. The ubiquitous notion of 'civil society' sometimes appears to be a platform for all those who want to reduce the welfare state to a mere minimum by loading responsibilities onto cheap volunteer work. Lastly, dementia-friendly communities must not turn into a middle-class project for well-situated families who are looking for new ways to get their elderly family members into a position of safety. There is a need for a braver spirit of opposition amongst those who are working to make dementia-friendly communities a reality. While we welcome and appreciate the approval offered by municipal authorities and mayors, we sometimes wish for a touch of piracy, with citizens boarding their communities and retaking their positions at the helm. Dementia-friendly communities must not be about conveniently exiling dementia from the open public arena into the invisible underground of local bourgeois communities. As we have tried to show in this chapter, instead of seeing dementia as a problem and asking what we can do about it, we need to start seeing dementia as an opportunity for change, and ask what it can do for us.

Note

1   We would like to thank Michael and Boka En for their help with the English version of this article.

References

Aktion Demenz (2008) Esslinger Aufruf. [Online] Available: www.aktion-demenz. de/besser-leben-mit-demenz/esslinger-aufruf.html (18 March 2013).

Anders, G. (1980) *Die Antiquiertheit des Menschen* (5th edn). Vol. 1. *Über die Seele im Zeitalter der zweiten industriellen Revolution.* Munich: C.H. Beck.

Baumann, Z. (2007) *Consuming Life.* Cambridge: Polity Press.

Bindé, J. (2010) 'Die Tyrannei der Dringlichkeit'. In: *Nano.Gen.Tech. Wie wollen wir leben?*, Paris: Edition Le Monde diplomatique, 38–44.

Gronemeyer, R. and Wißmann, P. (2008) *Demenz und Zivilgesellschaft – eine Streitschrift.* Frankfurt am Main: Mabuse-Verlag.

Gronemeyer, R. et al. (eds) (2007) Demenz und Kommune. [Online] Available: *www.aktion-demenz.de/images/stories/pdf/aktion_demenz08.pdf* (18 March 2013).

Jurk, C. (2012) *Menschen mit Demenz in der Kommune.* Evaluation von 12 Praxisprojekten der zweiten Ausschreibungsphase. Wiesbaden, 38–39.

Kreutzner, G. and Rothe, V. (eds) (2009) Aufbruch – In unserer Kommune: Gemeinsam für ein besseres Leben mit Demenz. [Online] Available: www.aktion-demenz.de/images/stories/aktion_demenz_screen.pdf (18 March 2013).

Peuckert, R. (2012) *Familienformen im sozialen Wandel.* Wiesbaden: VS Verlag für Sozialwissenschaften.

Philipp-Metzen, H.E. (2008) *Die Enkelgeneration im ambulanten Pflegesetting bei Demenz: Ergebnisse einer lebensweltorientierten Studie.* Wiesbaden: VS Verlag für Sozialwissenschaften.

Robert Bosch Stiftung (2007) *Gemeinsam für ein besseres Leben mit Demenz.* 7 Bände. Bern: Hans Huber Verlag.

Shiva, V. (2009) 'Die Krise wird uns zur ökologischen Landwirtschaft zwingen.' In G. von Lüpke, *Zukunft entsteht aus der Krise,* Munich: Riemann-Verlag.

Siegrist, J. (2010) 'Erfolgreich altern.' In Nano.Gen.Tech. Wie wollen wir leben?, Paris: Edition Le Monde diplomatique, 88–94.

Stadt Arnsberg (2011) Arnsberger 'Lern-Werkstatt' Demenz – Handbuch für Kommunen. [Online] Available: www.projekt-demenz-arnsberg.de/cms/upload/docs/PDA_Handbuch_weblinksDS.pdf (18 March 2013).

14 On the way to a Caring Community?

The German debate

Thomas Klie

'We are concerned about the care' – care we will receive whenever we are in need of it. We cannot rely on our families when we grow old nor be certain that nursing homes promise a good life. What age really means is to need protection. When looking at one's own vulnerability, age is a consideration for all of us. The issue of care is relevant for us all. And both parts, carers and people in need of care, need support because caring is not only a question of age. Therefore the issue of welfare worries mayors and citizens alike. Our cities and communities grow smaller and the general standard of living is facing challenges. Young families worry about the child-friendly aspects of our culture and the infrastructure that is so essential for growth and increasingly important for achieving a work–life balance. Meanwhile, we are concerned about the quality of life for seriously ill and dying individuals in a society in which death increasingly takes place in institutions. To live and to die, where one belongs (Dörner, 2007) is a profound wish shared by many people, yet for this to be fulfilled we have to look at the fundamental aspects of our cultural, infrastructural, financial, and technical situation.

The concept of a *Caring Community* is booming. But what is really behind it all? Is it merely a programme that helps to save on public spending, or is it nothing more than a new slogan? Does it mean taking advantage of the resource of 'commitment'? Even semantically, there are many variations upon this basic theme. There is, for example, talk of *Care-Taking Communes*, *Care-Taking Communities* or *Communities of Responsibility*. The sphere of activity and subject areas in which a Caring Community can be developed are diverse: Caring communes (or communities) in essence are concerned about sustainability, children, integration, values and spirituality, towards *others*, towards the sick and the dying and the bereaved. This approach is being picked up not only at local levels but also in schools, universities and in companies – especially in the United States. Also one can find the term in programmes of coordinated care: especially when it comes to the reconstruction of social contexts. These are related to so-called *compassionate communities* (Kellehear, 2005), a term to be found in discussions on health policy and palliative care. For some, though, the concept arouses suspicion: Is the state pulling away from its responsibility and wishing to revive the traditional role of women? Is this concept of care inappropriate for a late modern society that is reliant on the individual (Klie, 2014a), or do we need a new approach?

The Caring Community in the context of age

We live in a society of longevity, in which issues of intergenerational solidarity are on the agenda and anchored in our social awareness – with all the ambivalences attendant upon it. The concept of care can help to raise awareness even for smaller issues of concern – and help to reflect upon the requirements and meanings associated with these. In this context, older people worry about future generations and the potential considerable financial burden placed on them, being expected to provide financial input into the current system of care. The annual intergenerational transfers of older people exceed the governmental welfare spending that is needed for the younger ones in Germany – spending on basic security in old age. Meanwhile, older people play a significant role in terms of caring for grandchildren. In many neighbourhoods millions of older people are caring for future generations and within their age group are providing mutual support, monitoring and maintenance, which would be unthinkable without their contribution.

Who will take care of me when I am in need of it? According to the so-called *Sorgenbarometer* (Worry Barometer) (Schneyink, 2012), the issue of care for the elderly has top priority. The younger generation is very much aware of future issues, observing the current social security system and realizing that no real security in old age is likely to be provided for them. The question of how we can care for one another concerns many people, on an individual, collective and political level. In this respect, the question arises: Can the welfare state keep its original promises?

From the perspective of gerontology, we speak of a 'deinstitutionalization of age' and the diverse society of the elderly, or *'bunte Altersgesellschaft'* (Rosenmayr, 1994). Taking into account the opportunities and impositions upon one's own life in old age, we live in a society of longevity and have to shape our lives to fit those circumstances, both individually and collectively. Care also entails caring for oneself and one's own old age. We have many options for a good life in old age, if we truly have the capabilities to do so. Many older people are aware of their options in terms of housing, voluntary commitment, consumption and leisure, and realize that it is important to take precautions, not only with regard to our own health, but also in social, mental and spiritual terms. One of the most interesting results of interdisciplinary research in gerontology is the realization that the predictors of life expectancy are not primarily found in high blood pressure and cholesterol levels, but in the quality of our social networks. This brings a precautionary dimension into the spotlight, as our understanding of care is not (primarily) the synthetic screening of insurance companies, but the focus on social networks. To care for oneself thus mainly means to care for others. Here it is best to adopt Hannah Arendt's concept of co-responsibility (Arendt, 2013): The issues older people are concerned with – according to the results of a study by Andreas Kruse (2014) – do not primarily refer to health, but to the welfare of others. This also applies to young people, who feel similarly that relationships with others are highly significant. The opportunities and burdens of one's own life are embedded in relationships and the responsibility that comes with this. Does this fit into a postmodern society, with its individualism, its benefit considerations and its more pragmatic relationships?

The issue of care is one that touches everyone. This becomes abundantly clear simply by reflecting upon Caring Communities and age. Our notions of intergenerational relationships and life in old age are always embedded in a context of responsibility – and not at all in a conflict-free concept of social interaction. In the 6th Report on the Elderly (BMFSFJ, 2010) four anthropological models for ageing and age were formulated that give Caring Communities an anthropological basis: independence, meaning that one has the freedom to shape one's own life, self-responsibility (and here not a neoliberal welfare-state concept but in a profound anthropological sense), co-responsibility that seeks happiness not only within oneself, but is focused on others and on public spaces, as well as accepting dependency on others in return. This may be hard to comprehend, but it forms the basis for a society that is aware of our mutual responsibility for each other.

Caring Community in the context of family

An indication for the importance of a Caring Community is the family. We understand the importance of intergenerational relationships and at the same time are witnessing dramatic changes in modern family structures. The concept of family is fundamental to our culture, and to the moral framework that underpins it, in the sense of a transfer of commitments through the generations. The latter are, as Frank Schulz-Nieswandt puts it, highly effective and significant in both moral and economic respects (Schulz-Nieswandt, 2006). The 8th Family Report deals with the subject of the compatibility of family, work and care with a focus on time management. This will be the key issue of Caring Communities.

Both having responsibility for others and social interaction demand a great deal of our available time. Nowadays, time is one of our most precious commodities and the accelerating rate of extension of working hours and availability for work mean that limited time remains for social interaction, so that there is no real time to exercise care activities. But when it comes to the compatibility of work and time policy it is worth looking to other European countries. How is it possible that for example Norway and Sweden have a highly developed social system and at the same time enough time to care, which means time for duties within the family – and this is true for both genders. An explanation may be found in the relationship between social infrastructure and relatively rigid working hours. The legal, but even more the cultural, limitation placed upon working hours seems to be a significant factor. The Scandinavian countries offer us an example by which volunteering is positively correlated with an active welfare state. Time policy and the compatibility of education and care are questions that are highly relevant for Caring Communities in the context of family policy. Without linking to such issues, the Caring Community model remains merely appellative.

The concept of care

Revisiting the notion of *concern* may seem rather fussy and old fashioned. Others react aversely to what may be seen semantically as a backwards step towards a more traditional ideology of family, and the de-professionalization and romanticizing of mutual solidarity. In Germany, the term *concern* has an enduring patriarchal and authoritarian undertone. Today, the concept of *concern* is becoming relevant again. I prefer to describe *concern* as a 'progressive and compassionate way of taking on responsibility for oneself and others'. Albert Camus calls it: 'The simple "worry" is the beginning of all' (Camus, 2013). For Camus, to care for others and their happiness is the central dimension of human existence. A willingness and interest to shape society from the bottom up are essential motives for becoming involved. This sense of co-responsibility that motivates citizens has been an issue in studies of voluntary activities (Gensicke and Geiss, 2010). *Concern* refers to the immediate social environment: in relation to family, friends and neighbours (social proximity) and to society.

The rediscovery of a *prima vista* old-fashioned concept of *concern* expounds the problem of a more economics-oriented approach and with it the downgrading of people into customers, and into recipients of quality-assured services. Empathy and anticipatory responsibility mean so much more than the DIN ISO standardization of quality. The rediscovery of *concern* in civic and political discourse can trigger important processes of reflection on the logic underpinning the welfare state. Herein lies its quality of productive irritation.

Many citizens care about 'Care'. Many have doubts over whether they will be cared for when they cannot cope on their own any more. Care homes have turned into a bugbear and only 1 per cent of German citizens 'wish' to die in a hospital. On the other hand, they do not want to be a burden to their relatives. People are afraid of inadequate provision, despite increasing quality assurances and controls in and around homes. A particular contemporary concern is for one's own dignity and identity when it comes to serious illness and care. 'That's not how I want to end': as a 'nursing case', or as a 'demented idiot'. A willingness to book a one-way ticket to Zurich is increasing, and two-thirds of the German population support the legalization of assisted suicide. Being existentially reliant on the help of others and no longer being a successful person who is in control is an insult to the self-determined and autonomous self-image of people in our societies.

Community

The idea of the Caring Community is that of a collective. Yet although there is talk of communities who *care*, what exactly do we mean by this? Sometimes, Caring Communities are equated with a modern welfare mix, the interaction of government, service providers, neighbourhoods and families. In the example of the Freiburg model for group homes for people with dementia, people speak of *shared responsibilities*; a concept and practice that enable healthcare professionals, family members and public authorities to work together on a synergistic and co-productive level. Shared responsibility and a welfare mix do not however necessarily mean that this takes the form of a community, yet it requires the existence of a community. Shared responsibility is based on intelligent interaction, a culture of understanding and negotiation and the economic efficiency of such an arrangement. Community means a great deal more than welfare-based arrangements. Communities are characterized by belonging, common values and reciprocity.

We know that communities take diverse forms, including the family, also in a familial–sociological sense, which extends beyond blood ties, neighbourhoods, friends, forms of self-organization and association, and religious communities, with their spiritual focus. For many people with a migration background, it is important to experience community and belonging within their faiths, to share values and to preserve their cultural identity. Religion is no longer connected to the place in which you live – *cuius regio, eius religio*. Nevertheless, religion-based commitment on a local level can promote solidarity structures, if they are open in this respect. The territorial context, formed by communes with their different levels, e.g. rural districts, boroughs and urban districts, is the arena where social collaboration and mutual responsibility are practised (Binkert and Klie, 2004). Even communities based on choice can be Caring Communities. Where we feel that we belong to remains our decision and depends on the openness of the communities in question, from the welcoming culture in neighbourhoods, to the openness of peer groups, religious groups and churches. Responsibility and trust are the foundation of a sustainable society. It is within these small spheres of life that belonging and social attention matter, and they do so not by technically observing or monitoring, but by sharing values and a sense of security with the central notion of trust and responsibility. The subsidiary function of the state is to promote the necessary conditions that enable the creation and maintenance of communities. The state has to be active wherever community life is not functioning on its own or is at risk.

Subsidiarity

The question of the traditional principles of subsidiarity is raised particularly where we reflect upon the state and the role model this plays for Caring Communities. What can we do in a postmodern society with the principle of subsidiarity, and what do we mean by subsidiarity (Klie, 2014b)?

Hans F. Zacher was the first German legal practitioner who habilitated in social law, for which reason he had to go to Switzerland, and he is seen as one of the key architects of our social law order. Even today, Hans Zacher (1968) sees subsidiarity as the guiding principle of the liberal welfare state. For him subsidiarity guarantees that social issues receive attention – in families, in neighbourhoods and other small units of self-organization, if necessary with governmental support. A subsidiary order can activate a variety of forces. Subsidiarity can create space for autonomy, self-responsibility and co-responsibility and brings oxygen to the entire system. Hans Zacher describes precisely how subsidiarity shapes our social legal doctrine, which is unfortunately being progressively weakened by the current social legislation law, even though subsidiarity is the principle of order and outcome at the same time. However, this requires that an overall task is distributed among a variety of actors and institutions that complement each other. It is not just about the distribution of quality assured financial services, but also the Social as a whole, the capability to care, that needs to be looked at and cannot be taken for granted in a postmodern society. The socio-political approach of welfare pluralism is significantly important here. This includes specifically the tasks related to care, that have been undertaken by a group of welfare professionals. Because of the increasing tendency to monetize the social sector and the decrease of traditional forms of community life, the social state has an obligation to make sure that civil society and the informal sector are able to make their contribution and do not get pushed back or exploited.

Simple images of concentric circles of responsibility do not really represent our postmodern, functionally differentiated society in an adequate way. More is required for social networks and self-organized citizens to collaborate with government bodies and institutions. It takes vibrant neighbourhoods that are such an important backup for all forms of social interaction. This requires appropriate resources and local skills, from nursery schools to local youth services to neighbourhood management. These maintenance bases could make an important contribution regarding the care of people with disabilities or nursing needs, yet they have only been able to achieve this in two federal states (Saarland and Rheinland-Pfalz). Local contexts offer a perfect setting for this interaction, both centralized (social benefits law) and decentralized (infrastructure). German cooperative federalism with its inherent finance problems and the increasingly competition-oriented social services, such as health insurance, impede social care politics. This also becomes evident in the approach of Caring Communities.

Patient care, Caring Communities and the subsidiarity principle are always embedded in the discourse of gender and justice. It is not possible to re-conceptualize the principle of subsidiarity without addressing gender issues. The distribution of tasks is still connected to a pre-modern role model, exemplified in the fiscal planning of healthcare insurance. The cultural challenge of demographics and social change lies in a fair and intelligent redistribution of care responsibilities in the field of gender and generation; without recourse to a familial revisionism, as Adalbert Evers (Evers and Olk, 1996) puts it. If this succeeds, then it will be an interesting project for field workers and for national discourse to negotiate justice and gender issues in relation to Caring Communities. Should this not happen, there is a danger that the traditional women's role will become revitalized, or a conservative symbolic policy is pursued, which does everything to distract from urgent social and socio-political reforms.

The subsidiarity principle not only affects social organization but reminds us that the basis of social policy is anthropology. It touches on important ethical dimensions of our society. The subsidiarity principle is not only a part of Catholic social teaching in a triad with the principles of personality and solidarity, but it builds on an anthropology of freedom and responsibility. For Heinz Bude (Bude and Böhnk, 2006), the subsidiarity principle is the ethical standard for social policy design. He asks whether our action is limited by subsidiarity-related caution, if we set the all-day school against non-profit recreational activities and initiatives. The decline of engagement amongst young people in all-day schools is quite obvious. Is this okay? Is it what we want? Can the initiative of parents be replaced by quality-assured care? Are a master's degree or professionalized services always required to diagnose the resilience progress of a child? This does not mean that there is something wrong with having a good standard of knowledge, especially regarding children who fail our school system or vice versa. But especially in this context, a degree of ethical caution is required. Flat-sharing versus nursing homes, quality-assured service versus self-organization: what is the nature of the current dispute in Southern Germany about the quality management of home care? The confidence of social policy makers in welfare concepts and hybrid organizations of organization is currently low (cf. Evers, 2005; Evers et al., 2002). The only involvement of the state in coping with expanding responsibility concerns controlling institutions. Yet does such control really help? It is now well known that excellently run homes or all the annual inspections cannot prevent massive human rights violations from occurring. For Bude, welfare institutions should prove that their interventions do not contradict the principles of subsidiarity – at least in the context of regional and local planning.

If we try to revise the concept of subsidiarity in the context of the discussions surrounding Caring Community, it is advisable to follow Baumgartner and Korff (1999), who raised the question back in 1999, of how the tasks of joint support, which is relevant at all levels of society, can be solved using subsidiarity. In the spirit of subsidiarity, 'the diversity of social units extending from the ground up should be respected, preserved, and strengthened where it proves more competent than what is delivered by a higher-level social control system'.

This would be subsidiarity directed towards a modern society. Unlike pre-modern societies with their clear assignment of roles in families and society, it is characteristic of a modern society that there is a variety of actors and arrangements that require a pluralistic form of subsidiarity and an active social policy. The welfare state correlates with the pre-modern and modern varieties of subsidiarity. In pre-modern societies, traditional solidarity emanates from families, while in modern societies, it is civil society that increasingly follows subsidiarity principles. In order to manifest them in the culture and attitudes of citizens, a sociogenesis and psychogenesis are required in parallel, which is why anthropology and civilization are so important and have to be reclaimed in order to build a basis for social policy.

Subsidiarity is no longer considered to be a primarily formal principle that binds state action along the lines of charities rather than municipalities. Nor is it primarily a matter of creating cost-effective solutions to social problems. According to Emmanuel Levinas (1998), the ethics of subsidiarity are enshrined in the 'quality of unlimited liability', which Heinz Bude states has its origins in the familial experience, but which must prove itself according to relations that exist to the foreigner next door. This definition reveals the anthropological, almost religious and humanistic quality of the subsidiarity principle, because 'the quality of unlimited responsibility' has no rational calculus. In cultural mediation, these principles of responsibility are essential for subsidiarity and social interaction, for which reason socialization plays a central role. If we do not recognize their importance for our culture and learn how to apply them early enough, market logic in the social sector, welfare state expectations, the power structures of social administration, which increasingly prepare themselves for the failure of their regulatory efforts, are all able to damage the foundation of subsidiarity. So what does a social order, applied in subsidiarity, mean in words? Heinz Bude (Bude and Böhnk, 2006) distinguishes three levels:

- a person that is autonomous and takes personal initiative: 'Live your own life!'
- the strong and supporting social system: 'Look after your neighbour!'
- the ensuring and regulating state: 'Have the overview and look at the general picture!'

Local communities and a society of responsibility

When local communities talk about a *Society of Responsibility*, this does not refer to the operation of general standards of distribution in order to participate in quality-assured services in the logic of an economic approach to social work. It refers in fact – as Marianne Heimbach-Steins (2007) argues – to the locations and initiatives of welfare responsibility and the balancing act of solidarity undertaken in society as a whole. The social state needs to establish a framework design and local options for action. There are numerous recommendations for a new family policy and a necessary re-municipalization:

- from the study 'Network: Reshape the Social System' (SONG, 2009)
- from a cooperative study by the German Foundation for the Care of the Elderly (*Kuratorium Deutsche Altershilfe* – KDA) together with the Friedrich Ebert Foundation (FES and KDA, 2013), which addresses precisely these thoughts and relationships
- from a paper supported by the Robert Bosch Foundation on the structural reform of care and participation (Hoberg et al., 2013).

Overall, the socio-political re-evaluation of local authorities plays a major role in the context of Caring Communities. The responsibility for infrastructure lies in the hands of local authorities and does so in such a way that communities are the beneficiaries of social investments. The de facto dominance of central policy making in performance right across national agencies has taken hold in many areas and has marginalized communities in their ability and willingness to manage local affairs. This is true for Caring Communities, the aim of which is to turn communities into places for living the good life, with good housing facilities and the inclusion of older people – and those who are ill or disabled. In a society of longevity and demographic change, the capacity of a community to be an inclusive one is, alongside economic prosperity, an essential factor for the advantage of proximity.

Politically speaking, a borough is constituted as the smallest administrative authority in the state as well as in a cooperative, according to Article 28 of the German constitution. Having said this, one has to consider that boroughs, local authorities, city districts or neighbourhoods are all municipality levels with different structures, competencies and spaces of identification. Schulz-Nieswandt's concept of the *Inclusion Community* is helpful when examining potential directions of Caring Communities. Within an Inclusion Community, a community forms a stronger collaborative and interpersonal cohesion. Life is directed toward others: in terms of social attention, neighbourly support, cooperative forms of managing common life and accepting disparity and diversity. Schulz-Nieswandt's vision concerns the cooperative nature of *polity* under modern conditions of personal authenticity (Schulz-Nieswandt, 2013). The community benefits from being a legal association on the basis of reciprocity and on the anthropological condition of giving and receiving.

But an approach such as this creates a number of challenges for local authorities. These include:

- overcoming the logic of the economization of all areas of life,
- overcoming an anachronistic romantic model of family,
- showing a new hospitality towards *homo patiens* (as a willingness to give and share with strangers and by overcoming fear, distance, disgust and other forms of differentiation),
- showing openness to the building of cooperatives in response to conditions in the field (public-sector service provision),
- the development of an innovation culture (guiding principles, structures, skills).

Whether such a substantial re-municipalization can succeed is not certain because not all local authorities are willing and able to do so. Their starting positions – culturally, politically and financially – differ greatly. The response of the Caring Communities model in different political spheres and among large parts of the population, the need to design a new preventive and caring social policy and to not surrender to the challenges of demographic change, are all factors that give the model a certain potential capacity.

In studies on urban demography planning, the idea of cooperatives and the productive development of 'care and concern' are highly attractive, with many local potentials. The programme 'Active in Old Age' (BMFSFJ, 2009) has made this visible in several hundred municipalities in Germany. The central importance of the participation and involvement in local social development has already been mentioned. These local developments differ in the way in which municipal authorities open up to the demographic and social changes. For Schulz-Nieswandt (2013) the municipalities can be divided into various types: the *innovative type* is already on the way to achieving positive change, the *disoriented, helpless type* is somewhat disoriented but ready to change, the *depressive type* only sees a bleak future and finds it difficult to accept help and the *ignorant type* is adhering to a know-it-all attitude. Depending on which type of municipal approach we encounter, we will find different conditions of living. The promotion of Caring Communities is thus embedded in a broad-based community development programme. It is no coincidence that KGSt (Germany's largest local government think tank) has a strong focus on the topic of civic community. Also, the Social City programme supports a culture of innovation in many quarters: the intertwining of federal political incentive structures with local development potential is an essential indicator of success for a policy that is devoted to the mission statement for Caring Communities.

Conclusion

The mission statement of the Caring Community concept triggers controversy in Germany. For some it carries the problematic conservative features of a backward approach to family policy and a romanticized notion of

208   *Thomas Klie*

neighbourhoods and districts in modern societies. What is intended to supply the social interaction? It reduces the duties of the welfare state and subordinates citizens to the dictate of optimization – now also in terms of commitment and concern. For others, the model provides a perspective for a necessary realignment of social policy in times of demographic and social change. If these new developments are really desired then this will have major consequences for the architecture of our 'care policies'. In any case, the model raises fundamental anthropological questions: What significance does the modern human being give to the care of others in a postmodern society? To find that out, it is worth arguing – in Germany and in many other countries.

References

Arendt, H. (2013) *Vita activa oder Vom tätigen Leben* (13th edn). München: Piper.
Baumgartner, A. and Korff, W. (1999) Sozialprinzipien als ethische Baugesetzlichkeiten moderner Gesellschaft: Personalität, Solidarität und Subsidiarität. In W. Korff et al. (eds) *Handbuch der Wirtschaftsethik (Vol. 1): Verhältnisbestimmung von Wirtschaft und Ethik*. Gütersloh: Gütersloher Verlags-Haus, 225–237.
Blinkert, B. and Klie, T. (2004) *Solidarität in Gefahr. Pflegebereitschaft und Pflegebedarfsentwicklung im demografischen und sozialen Wandel. Die 'Kasseler Studie'*. Hannover: Vincentz Network.
Bude, H. and Böhnke, P. (2006) *Das Problem der Exklusion*. Hamburg: Hamburger Edition.
Bundesministerium für Familie, Senioren, Frauen und Jugend (BMFSFJ) (2009) *Mitgestalten und mitentscheiden. Das Programm 'Aktiv im Alter'*. Online: www. bmfsfj.de/ Redaktion BMFSFJ/Broschuerenstelle/Pdf-Anlagen/mitgestalten-mitentscheiden,property= pdf, bereich=bmfsfj, sprache=de, rwb=true.pdf (accessed 10 September 2014).
Bundesministerium für Familie, Senioren, Frauen und Jugend (BMFSFJ) (ed.) (2010) *Sechster Bericht zur Lage der älteren Generation in der Bundesrepublik Deutschland. Altersbilder in der Gesellschaft*. Deutscher Bundestag, Drucksache 17/3815. Online: www. bmfsfj.de/ RedaktionBMFSFJ/Abteilung3/Pdf-Anlagen/ bt-drucksache-sechster-altenbericht (accessed 21 July 2014).
Camus, A. (2013) *Der Mythos des Sisyphos* (16th edn). Reinbek bei Hamburg: Rowohlt.
Dörner, K. (2007) *Leben und sterben, wo ich hingehöre. Dritter Sozialraum und neues Hilfesystem*. Neumünster: Paranus-Verlag der Brücke Neumünster.
Evers, A. (2005) Mixed welfare systems and hybrid organizations. Changes the governance and provision of social services. *International Journal of Public Administration* 28: 737–748.
Evers, A. and Olk, T. (eds) (1996) *Wohlfahrtspluralismus. Vom Wohlfahrtsstaat zur Wohlfahrtsgesellschaft*. Opladen: Westdeutscher Verlag.
Evers, A., Rauch, U. and Stitz, U. (2002) *Von öffentlichen Einrichtungen zu sozialen Unternehmen. Hybride Organisationsformen im Bereich sozialer Dienstleistungen*. Eine Studie der Hans-Böckler-Stiftung. Online: www.worldcat.org/ oclc/231927218 (accessed 21 July 2014).

Friedrich-Ebert-Stiftung (FES) and Kuratorium Deutsche Altershilfe (KDA) (eds) (2013) *Gute Pflege vor Ort. Das Recht auf ein eigenständiges Leben im Alter. WISO Diskurs.* Online: http://library.fes.de/pdf-files/wiso/10170.pdf (accessed 21 July 2014).

Gensicke, T. and Geiss, S. (2010) *Hauptbericht des Freiwilligensurveys 2009.* Zivilgesellschaft, soziales Kapital und freiwilliges Engagement in Deutschland 1999–2004–2009. TNS Infratest Sozialforschung, München. Online: www.bmfsfj.de/RedaktionBMFSFJ/Broschuerenstelle/Pdf-Anlagen/3._20Freiwilligensurvey-Hauptbericht, property=pdf,bereich=bmfsfj,sprache=de,rwb=true.pdf (accessed 21 July 2014).

Heimbach-Steins, M. (2007) Wohlfahrtsverantwortung. Ansätze zu einer sozialethischen Kriteriologie für die Verhältnisbestimmung von Sozialstaat und freier Wohlfahrtspflege. In M. Dabrowski and J. Wolf (eds) *Aufgaben und Grenzen des Sozialstaats.* Paderborn: Schöningh Verlag, 9–42.

Hoberg, R., Klie, T. and Künzel, G. (2013) *Strukturreform Pflege und Teilhabe.* Extended version. Freiburg: FEL Verlag.

Kellehear, A. (2005) *Compassionate Cities. Public Health and End-of-Life Care.* London: Routledge.

Klie, T. (2014a) *Wen kümmern die Alten? Auf dem Weg in eine sorgende Gesellschaft.* München: Pattloch.

Klie, T. (2014b) Subsidiarität in der postmodernen Gesellschaft: Ein Sicherheitsversprechen? In H. Hoch and P. Zoche (eds) *Zivile Sicherheit. Schriften zum Fachdialog Sicherheitsforschung* (Vol. 8). Berlin: LIT Verlag, 355–381.

Kruse, A. (2014) Der Ältesten Rat. Generali Hochaltrigenstudie: *Teilhabe im hohen Alter.* Eine Erhebung des Instituts für Gerontologie der Universität Heidelberg mit der Unterstützung des Generali Zukunftsfonds. Online: www.uni-heidelberg.de/md/presse/ news2014/generali_hochaltrigenstudie.pdf (accessed 21 July 2014).

Levinas, E. (1998) *Éthique comme philosophie première.* Paris: Éditions Payot et Rivages.

Netzwerk Soziales neu gestalten (SONG) (2009) *Lebensräume zum Älterwerden – Für ein neues Miteinander im Quartier.* Online: www.bertelsmann-stiftung.de/cps/rde/xbcr/SID-B411AE7C-39C94787/bst/xcms_bst_dms_27817_27818_2.pdf (accessed 21 July 2014).

Rosenmayr, L. (1994) Altersgesellschaft – bunte Gesellschaft? Soziologische Analyse als Beitrag zur politischen Orientierung. In A. Evers, K. Leichsenring and B. Marin (eds) *Die Zukunft des Alterns. Sozialpolitik für das Dritte Lebensalter.* Wien: Bundesministerium für Arbeit und Soziales, 27–76.

Schneyink, D. (2012) *Stern-Sorgenbarometer. Die Rückkehr der 'German Angst'.* Online: www.stern.de/politik/deutschland/stern-sorgenbarometer-die-rueckkehr-der-german-angst-1907249.html (accessed 21 July 2014).

Schulz-Nieswandt, F. (2006) *Sozialpolitik und Alter. Grundriss Gerontologie* (Vol. 5). Stuttgart: Kohlhammer.

Schulz–Nieswandt, F. (2013) *Der leidende Mensch in der Gemeinde als Hilfs- und Rechtsgenossenschaft.* Berlin: Duncker & Humblot.

Zacher, H. (1968) *Sozialpolitik und Menschenrechte in der Bundesrepublik Deutschland.* München: Olzog.

Index